GOING VEGAN

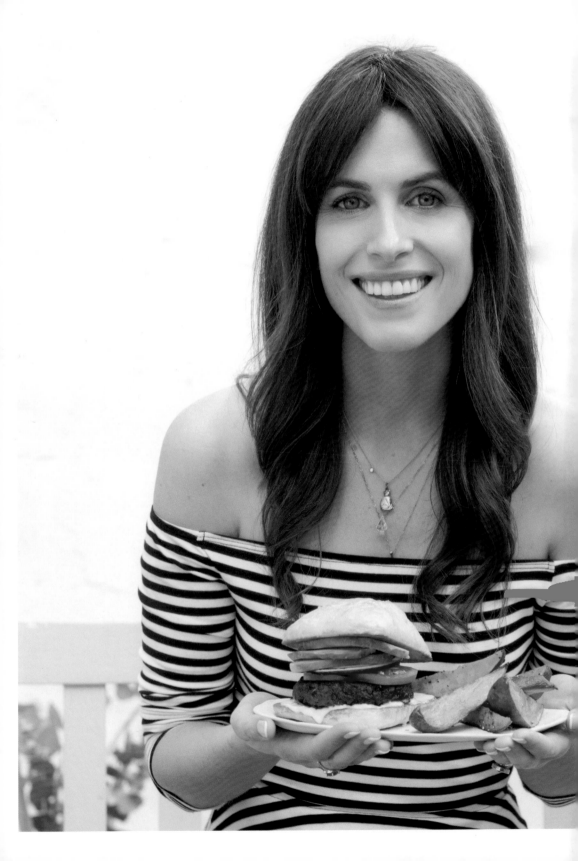

GOING VEGAN

A Gentle Introduction to
A PLANT-BASED DIET

HOLLY WHITE

Skyhorse Publishing

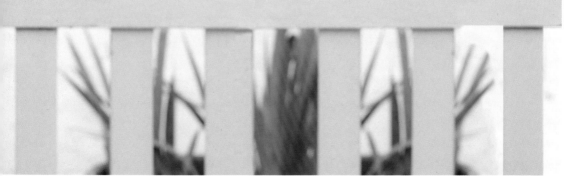

Originally published by Gill Books, Hume Avenue, Park West, Dublin 12, www.gillbooks.ie

Gill Books is an imprint of M.H. Gill and Co.

© Holly White 2018

Skyhorse Publishing books may be purchased in bulk at special discounts for sales promotion, corporate gifts, fund-raising, or educational purposes. Special editions can also be created to specifications. For details, contact the Special Sales Department, Skyhorse Publishing, 307 West 36th Street, 11th Floor, New York, NY 10018 or info@skyhorsepublishing.com.

Skyhorse® and Skyhorse Publishing® are registered trademarks of Skyhorse Publishing, Inc.®, a Delaware corporation.

Visit our website at www.skyhorsepublishing.com.

10 9 8 7 6 5 4 3 2 1

Library of Congress Cataloging-in-Publication Data is available on file.

Cover design by Mona Lin
Designed by www.grahamthew.com
Structural Editor: Kristen Jensen
Proofread by Jane Rogers
Indexed by Eileen O'Neill
Photography by Leo Byrne Photography
Food Styling by Charlotte O'Connell

Print ISBN: 978-1-5107-5283-2
Ebook ISBN: 978-1-5107-5284-9

Printed in China

CONTENTS

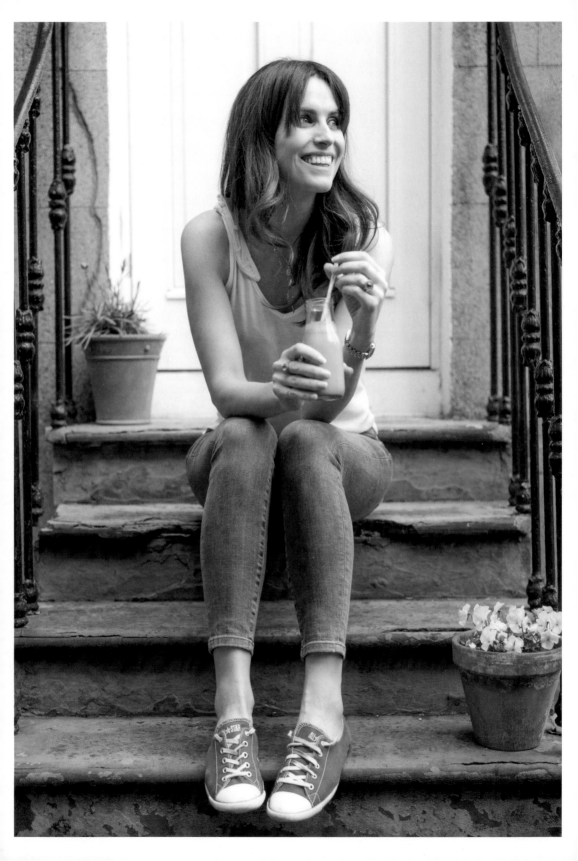

INTRODUCTION

AS I'M SITTING HERE writing with my deadline approaching, it's nearly three in the morning and I feel a little isolated from the rest of the world. It reminds me of the feeling I had when I first attempted to go vegan. I was a student in Trinity College in a course that I would later drop out of to pursue a totally different pathway.

I wanted to try eating a vegan diet, but while my friends went to the dining hall, I went – often alone and a little embarrassed – into town to try to find something, anything, that would tide me over. In those days my options were limited and I knew nothing about vegan proteins, fermentation, sprouting, nut milks or juicing.

Within a couple of weeks, I gave up.

When I turned 30 I went through the slightly clichéd re-evaluation of my life. Without even being consciously aware of what was happening, I noticed myself bookmarking nearly every vegan recipe that caught my eye. Something in me almost begged me to give it another try.

Around this time I watched a few documentaries, such as *Forks Over Knives*, *Earthlings*, *Before the Flood* and *Cowspiracy* (which is produced by eco-warrior Leonardo DiCaprio). Before I saw these films, I hadn't made the connection between what I was eating and the conditions – and the death – that were necessary to get meat to my table.

I wanted to be part of a positive social change but had no clue how I could do that. I gradually realised that by reducing animal proteins in my diet, ensuring that all my beauty products and make-up were cruelty-free and reducing single-use plastics, I could have a fundamental impact on the environment. It's estimated that by adopting a plant-based diet, you save 1,100 gallons of water, 30 square feet of forested land, 20lb CO_2 equivalent and one animal's life every single day. There's no doubt that switching to a vegan diet will be challenging, as eating meat, fish and dairy is ingrained in our way of life, but understanding the difference you're making by adopting a vegan diet is very rewarding.

On a more practical level, I had to re-educate myself entirely on what and how to eat. For the first year I lived off energy balls, pasta and tomato sauce, sweet potato fries and lots of hummus. Once I knew I was committed to this lifestyle, I started craving a wider variety of foods. I wanted to create the kind of satiating, beautiful and, most important, nourishing meals that would make people eager for invitations to dinner.

As a result of the way I eat now, I feel better in my thirties than I ever did in my twenties. Even on a simple outward level, my skin is clearer and in better condition now than it was 10 years ago. The ruddiness and red patches disappeared from my complexion within six weeks of cutting out red meat and dairy and my weight maintains itself in a way I wouldn't have thought possible before.

I have gone on to complete extensive vegan chef training both in Ireland and abroad and I now share recipes on my blog, host events and do demonstrations at festivals and on television. Not a day goes by that I don't get a positive message on my social media channels regarding a recipe, a recommendation or someone sharing a tip and it amazes me how something that was initially so isolating has now come full circle and created a wonderful community.

The past few years have opened my mind and broadened my palate in ways I never thought possible. People often ask me if I miss certain things, but I feel that I eat a much wider variety of foods now than I ever did before. I've become passionate about good food and great flavours and sharing this with other people.

While I'm not a fan of dramatic changes or doing things just because they're trendy, there's no doubt that veganism is a big thing. Lots of people are committing to a diet without any animal products, and having gone through it all myself, I have a lot of experience with the challenges you will face. I cut out meat and chicken overnight but kept eating very small amounts of dairy and fish, mainly in social situations, for about six months. That worked for me, but I know that the idea of going vegan cold turkey is pretty dramatic.

Whether you're already vegan or just looking for interesting ways to integrate more vegetables and pulses into your diet, here are some of my tips for going vegan-ish, no matter what stage you're currently at.

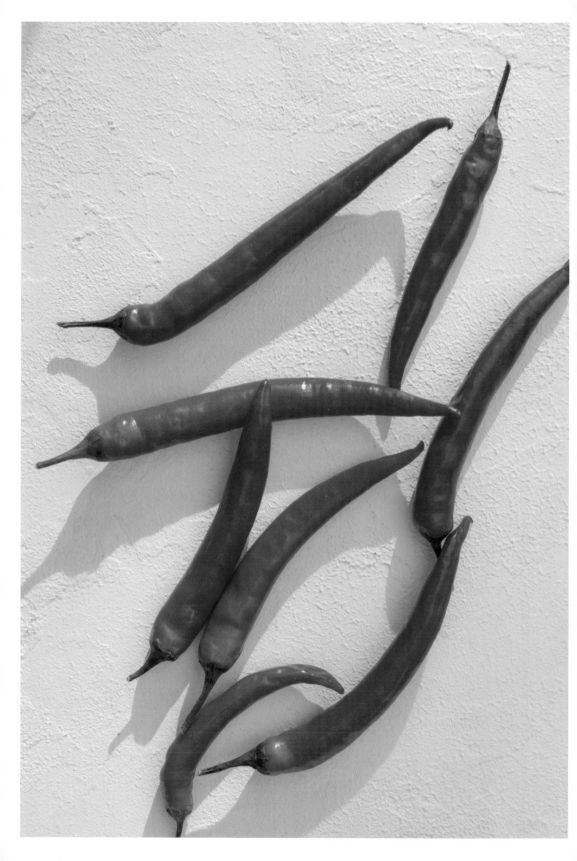

GOING VEGAN-ISH

THE FIRST RULE OF going vegan-ish is don't talk about going vegan-ish!

There are lots of internet memes about not needing to bother asking if someone is vegan, as they will tell you within a moment of meeting them, and they make me cringe. I advise people to wait a few months before telling anyone beyond their immediate friends and family that they're making changes to their lifestyle, as you need to see how you feel and what changes you want to make before being questioned about it.

It's really important that you figure out what kind of vegan lifestyle feels right to you. There are support groups (and also pressure groups) online, and while both serve a purpose, this is your journey and you are in the driver's seat. Whether it's a meatless Monday or an occasional dairy-free latte, there isn't a rule book for going vegan – it's your choice, and timeline, entirely.

You are doing this because you have chosen to and that it's your decision. However, you don't have the right to decide what other people choose to eat, bore them to tears by going on and on about your diet or give out to them for eating sausage rolls in front of you. Let people be drawn in by how good your food looks or how well you seem to be feeling.

KNOW WHO TO TRUST

I've done quite a lot of training and my bookshelves are heaving with cookbooks, but I'm not a professionally trained chef, doctor or nutritionist. I'm a home cook who is really passionate and curious about this way of eating. I've done a lot of personal research and I know what works for me.

Maintaining your health is a huge responsibility that you need to thoroughly research and evaluate to figure out what works for you, especially if you have a medical concern. The internet is rife with 'experts', but you should trust only qualified practitioners and reliable, qualified sources for medical advice or nutritional concerns. For example, I get my bloods tested annually to ensure I'm not anaemic and so that I can monitor any changes.

START SMALL

Veganism isn't just about food. I actually prefer the term 'plant-based' when talking about my diet, as veganism is an entire lifestyle that extends to excluding, as far as is possible and practicable, all forms of exploitation of and cruelty to animals for food, clothing or any other purpose. This means not going to zoos, wearing any form of leather or wool, or using any cosmetics that have animal ingredients.

Make the changes that feel easy at first. Go with your gut instinct – literally! – and try the recipes that you think sound the most appealing and delicious rather than diving headfirst into proteins you might have never seen, let alone eaten, before.

Bulking up a casserole with lentils in addition to whatever protein you have already included is an easy way to get used to integrating them into your diet. Making your own hummus versus buying it is another quick way to dip your toe into the vegan-ish world, as it's relatively cheap and you are probably already familiar with the taste of it. Most coffee shops will have dairy-free milks, so experimenting

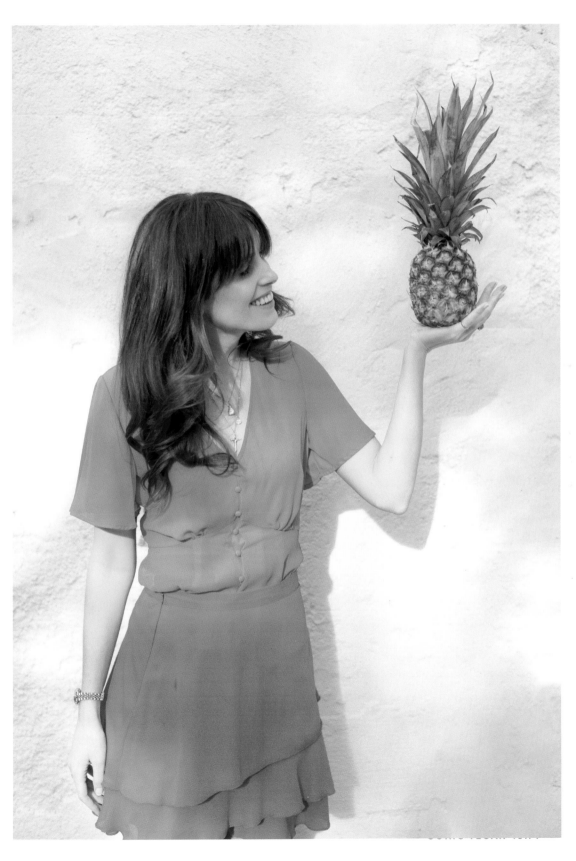

with them in your latte is a nice way to try the options without the expense of buying the produce and equipment needed to make them at home. At my demonstrations and events I make a range of food so that everyone can taste it and therefore see if they want to buy the raw ingredients to make things themselves at home afterwards.

Most important, I would advise you not to put any pressure on yourself and to do what feels right for you. While it's admirable that some people who go vegan commit to changing every element of their lifestyle, any step you choose to take is a positive one, even if it's just swapping to plant-based milk in your coffee or making sure your cosmetics are cruelty-free.

KEEPING PERSPECTIVE

It's important to have a sense of perspective. I eat this way by choice, as I don't have allergies or intolerances. My motto is to control what you can and otherwise go with the flow. If I'm out with friends or family and the food on offer isn't vegan, I quietly get on with it. While I won't eat meat, if a sauce or dish happens to have some dairy in it, I don't make too much of a fuss. At home I can control exactly what I eat, but I would never want to make someone who has kindly prepared a meal for me uncomfortable. If this is a change you have suddenly or recently made, don't expect that everyone around you will have a perfect vegan dish ready and waiting!

Rather than thinking about what you're missing out on, you need to focus on what you will gain, whether it's discovering a new restaurant or a new way to work around a menu, or even how to prep in advance so you're not starving.

While this might be controversial, I suggest that you try to be flexible about your strict veganism when eating out or in your friends' houses. If I were preparing food for a dinner party, getting a litany of dietary requests would drive me mad, so I try not to be that person.

Food is a social way to come together and the company and atmosphere take precedence for me. Don't use veganism as an excuse to isolate yourself. My stance on eating has always been to control what I can and go with the flow otherwise. Don't ruin a dinner party by sitting there with an empty plate making everyone feel awkward. Eat well beforehand, try what you like and don't draw too much attention to yourself. I always offer to bring a dish that I know I can eat and it makes me really happy when I see others enjoying it too!

For example, one evening my non-vegan brother invited me over for a casual dinner. I was experimenting with a vegan berry cheesecake I was due to demonstrate on TV, so I said I would bring dessert. He was delighted.

About half an hour later, realising that with a busy family and work life he probably wasn't thinking of preparing a vegan option, I asked him what he was serving. 'Spaghetti Bolognese,' was his speedy reply. I said that I would bring a lentil casserole for myself and anyone else who might like to try it.

Arriving at his house with both the dessert and a dinner option, I realised that this was the reality of the choice I have made for how I choose to eat. It's not always going to be easy for other people to accommodate you, nor should you always expect them to.

Leaving the house a few hours later with a scraped-clean pot and an empty cake tin was a lovely moment, though, as everyone had enjoyed the food I'd brought. So the moral of the story is never turn up to a party empty-handed.

EATING OUT

I'm continually amazed at how much effort restaurants will go to and how happy they are to accommodate a vegan diet as long as you give them notice. If you're making a booking it literally takes 30 seconds to let them know, and it will make your dining experience memorable for all the right reasons. If a group of us are going out I usually offer to book the restaurant, as that way I can let them know while making the reservation. Otherwise, I've put together some gorgeous meals from side dishes in lots of places. There's always an option, and remember, dining out is about the company first and foremost.

Be honest. I was at an event in a swanky Dublin restaurant and when I said I was vegan, the chef asked if I was 'actually vegan'. I was a bit confused, but then he told me that he had gone to extensive trouble to accommodate six vegans at a recent wedding, creating special dishes for them. All of them proceeded to order the fillet steak instead. If you want a night off from being vegan, that's fine, but it's disrespectful to ask a chef to prepare something special for you and then not follow through. They most likely won't go to the same effort again.

The very first question anyone will ask is, 'Where do you get your protein?' It's an important one to answer and also to understand.

Protein gives our bodies structure as part of our muscles and bones. It's also used for fighting infections, carrying oxygen, growth and repair.

It's easy for a vegan diet to meet the recommended dietary allowance for protein. Nearly all vegetables, beans, grains, nuts and seeds contain some, and often a lot of, protein. For example, gram for gram, lentils contain more protein than beef, but they are quite bland and need a little help to make them delicious. All will be revealed in the recipes!

A key thing to remember is that you must balance your meals. Initially I simply subtracted meat from my diet and existed off pasta and sweet potato fries and didn't feel great. Learning how to integrate key sources of vegan protein, such as beans, pulses, nuts and tofu, made a world of difference, but it took a bit of time and experimentation. I use a lot of superfoods in my cooking – say, raw cacao, which is a great source of iron and magnesium – not solely for taste, but for their nutritional benefits as well.

I'm not really into supplements, but I do have some good vegan protein powders and a liquid iron that I'll add to smoothies if I feel the need to during a busy period, if I'm doing a lot of exercise or just need a boost. There are lots of different brands, but I avoid the ones with synthetic-sounding flavours – toffee caramel marshmallow-flavoured protein is likely to be highly processed. I also get my blood tested regularly by my primary care physician. I would advise anyone who wants some reassurance to do the same and to track their results.

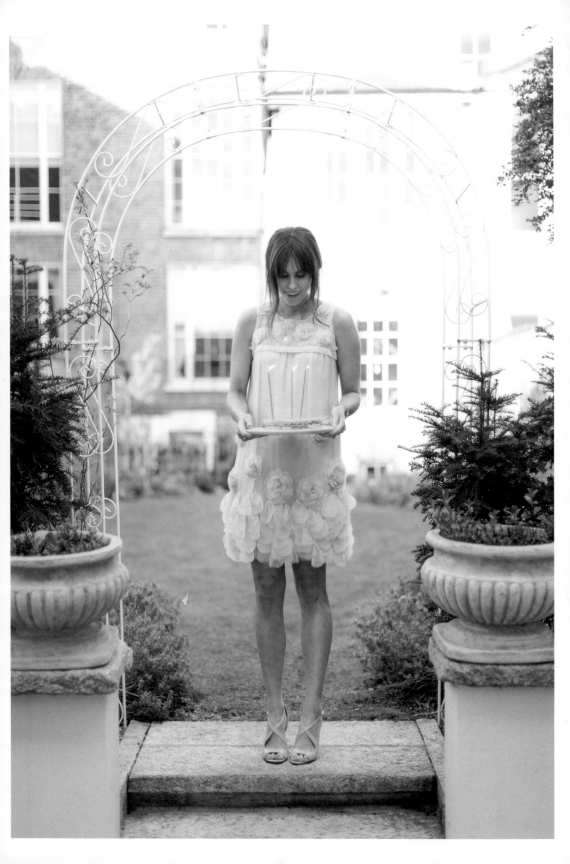

Pick a day of the week and batch cook some roasted veggies, brown rice, hummus, grilled tofu, curry paste and some energy balls and you'll be all set for a few days.

Bookmark recipes that catch your eye and store photos of them in a separate album on your phone so that they'll always be close to hand when you're shopping in the supermarket or need some inspiration.

BLENDED HOUSEHOLDS

One of the questions I am asked most often is how to deal with different diets in a busy household. I always suggest that you think of it in terms of food assembly. Having some chicken breast, mince or fish ready to add to a stir-fry or casserole transforms it. It's not about making separate dishes, it's about sectioning off a portion and adding meat to that if other people you are cooking for require it. Most of the flavours of the dish will likely be in the sauce, but if some members of your family are craving meat, make it an easy addition rather than an entirely different meal.

GIVE IN TO CRAVINGS

I think you should give in to your cravings, as sometimes if we think we can't have something, we can exaggerate its appeal in our minds. But you should also explore ways of trying textures and flavours you might be missing in your vegan-ish diet. For example, the first time I made my vegan shepherd's pie, I realised I had been missing something. The combination of the walnuts and the miso paste gives it a rich taste, and while I don't like heavy food, sometimes you want something really satisfying.

Every airline can accommodate a vegan diet as long as you let them know in advance. I always stock up on snacks and treats such as energy balls, chocolate, nuts, crisps or popcorn (my weakness!) to bring with me on the plane as well.

Do a bit of research online before you travel. There's nothing worse than a language barrier and a hungry tummy in the midday sun, so having somewhere mapped out for a meal in advance is ideal. Before I travel, I always ask my followers on social media to recommend places to eat or where to get a great coffee. Make sure to use a few hashtags of the place you're travelling to and hopefully you'll get some great recommendations.

Try to be flexible too and look at how things can be made vegan – for example, a pizza without cheese is vegan. Other places do vegan food effortlessly. I was in Thailand, I loved the food so much that within our first week I did a Thai cooking course.

If you're staying in self-catering accommodation and have cooking facilities, a quick shop in a local market for fresh bread, olive oil, fruit, nuts and vegetables is a great start. I'm a huge fan of antipasti and could eat back olives, artichokes, balsamic vinegar and olive oil with chunky bread and a glass of wine every night of the week, and thankfully I can find these in any local supermarket when I travel. You can buy small travel blenders or even email your host in advance to see if they have one so that you can make a smoothie, adding some vegan protein power if you like to set you up for the day.

HAVE FUN!

Not only is this food delicious, but it also has a phenomenally powerful effect on the environment – one of the most effective things an individual can do to lower their carbon footprint is to reduce their consumption or use of all animal products. Whether or not you're vegan, I hope you gain some inspiration from this book. Find your own path, have fun and enjoy every meal along the way. I hope this book shows you how truly delicious eating this way can be.

Lots of love,

Holly

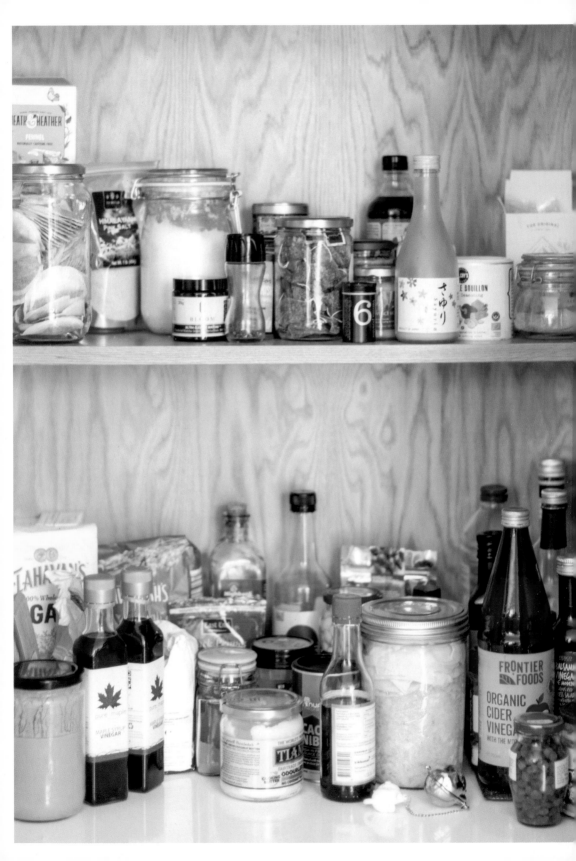

SHOP SMART

I DON'T HAVE ANY magic tricks up my sleeve or secret shops where I buy mystical ingredients. I live in the city centre and shop in my local supermarket for most of my ingredients, just in different aisles than I used to!

Your first supermarket shop or glance at a recipe might seem overwhelming or maybe just really unusual, but honestly, I don't spend huge amounts of time cooking or shopping now. I simply have a new normal, and I promise that if you allow for a short transition time and trust the recipes, it will all quickly become so much easier.

The great thing about a vegan diet is that except for your fruit and vegetables, it comprises a lot of cupboard staples that you can buy in bulk. About every six weeks or so I stock up the pantry with tinned and dried beans, olive oil, coconut milk, nuts, flour, oats, grains, rice, tinned tomatoes and spices, which form the backbone of the food I eat. I tend to do a light shop twice a week for fruit and vegetables, often going for what's on offer and in season, and build my meals around that.

I also find that my food bills are a lot cheaper than before. Some trips to the health food store are a little more expensive, but on a day-to-day basis, it's very affordable to eat this way. Look for offers on nuts and grains in supermarkets and build a relationship with your local health food store. While they might not have things like nutritional yeast or even a nut milk bag in-store, they can easily order them in. When I'm testing recipes and need large quantities of something – say, six tins of coconut milk during a yogurt experimentation phase – I'll ask for a discount and often find them to be very obliging. If you don't ask, you'll never know! But if you're ordering online, make sure that you are signed up to any loyalty schemes, which may save you some money.

A few slightly more niche items will elevate your cooking. In response to how we are all changing our diets you can buy most of these in supermarkets now, but if not, these are my health food store essentials. If you have an Asian market near you, it's a great place to stock up on spices, rice, tofu and miso pastes, often at very reasonable prices.

KEY INGREDIENTS

AGAVE SYRUP: My sweetener of choice is either agave syrup (also called agave nectar) or maple syrup. They both blend easily and are now readily available. There are different grades and strengths, i.e. agave comes in dark or light, so if you are swapping to a different brand, have a little taste to judge its sweetness. Agave can be used to sweeten tea and coffee too.

CACAO BUTTER: Cacao butter is a natural, meltable oil extracted from the cacao bean. It's the fat source used to give chocolate its alluring, melt-in-your-mouth, silky mouthfeel. It's brilliant for helping to stabilise desserts, as it melts and blends easily but is solid at room temperature.

CHIA SEEDS: When you cut out eggs, you have to look for other options as a binding agent when baking and chia seeds work really well. As a rough guide, mix 1 tablespoon of chia seeds with 3 tablespoons of filtered water and let sit for 15 minutes to gel to replace one egg in a recipe. They also naturally thicken smoothies and pancakes.

COCONUT AMINOS: Coconut aminos is a dark, rich, salty and slightly sweet sauce made from coconut sap. It resembles a light soy sauce or tamari, but it's soy-free and gluten-free, making it the perfect replacement for anyone avoiding soy and gluten. It's widely available in health food stores.

COCONUT MILK: When I call for coconut milk or cream in recipes, I'm referring to the tinned variety. When I mention coconut cream, I mean the creamy part that you can scoop from the top of a tin (see my tip on page 308 for how to do this). There are two grades of coconut milk: thick and thin. Thick coconut milk contains 20–22% fat, while thin coconut milk contains 5–7% fat. Look at the back of the tin to check which kind it is. Personally I never buy the low-fat variety, as I actually want the creamy part and because I feel it's less processed.

COCONUT OIL: Used both for cooking and in raw desserts, as it has a similar consistency to butter in that it solidifies at room temperature. When melted it blends easily, but when allowed to set it helps maintain firmness in desserts and chocolates.

HIMALAYAN PINK SALT: This is a naturally occurring salt that's high in minerals and has a beautiful pink colour. Himalayan pink salt contains over 84 minerals and trace elements, including calcium, magnesium, potassium, copper and iron.

LUCUMA POWDER: Lucuma powder is made from whole Peruvian lucuma fruit that has been dried at low temperatures and milled into a fine powder. This low-glycemic sweetener has a gorgeously rich caramel flavour and enhances desserts nutritionally.

MACA POWDER: Maca is a Peruvian plant that has been cultivated in the Andes Mountains for at least 3,000 years. It has a rich, sweet flavour that easily blends into desserts and smoothies.

MEDJOOL DATES: Not all dates are created equal. Medjool dates are more expensive, larger and more full of flavour than regular dates. Normal dates are perfectly fine in recipes, but you may find you need to add a few more to get a recipe to blend. If your dates are particularly tough or dry you will need to soften them in a cup of just-boiled water for about 15 minutes before use to save your blender. Always pit dates, and even if the packet says they are pitted, always double check, as the stones will not only ruin your recipe, but will damage your blender or food processor blade too.

MISO PASTE: This fermented soybean paste gives a fabulous umami boost to dishes and sauces. You can find it in the refrigerated section of health food shops or Asian markets.

NUTRITIONAL YEAST: This resembles fish food flakes, but don't underestimate it! It adds a cheesy flavour to sauces, soups, casseroles and stir-fries and is a vegan addiction. There are two varieties, so make sure that you get the one fortified with vitamin B12.

PROBIOTIC CAPSULES: A poor diet, taking antibiotics or simply the stresses and strains of modern living can disturb the delicate microfloral environment in the digestive tract. A probiotic capsule works to replenish 'friendly' gut bacteria, delivering up 42 billion live bacteria per capsule to both the small and large intestines. When adjusting your diet, I feel it's important to support and ocassionally supplement with a good probiotic. I always take them when travelling or if I have been unwell. They can also be used to cultivate yogurts and ferments, which is why I use them in some of my recipes.

RAW APPLE CIDER VINEGAR: This has a live fermented culture in it, called the mother, which is considered to be highly beneficial. It has an incredibly sharp tang that I love to use in dressings. Raw apple cider vinegar will look cloudy at the base of the bottle; check that the label says it includes the mother. Once I got a bit more into fermentation and learned about how incredible raw apple

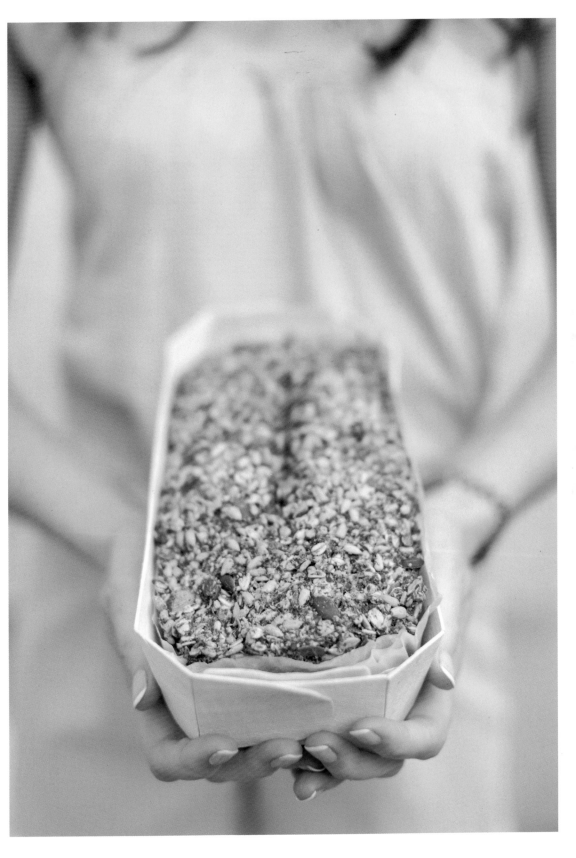

cider vinegar is, I wanted to use it as often as possible. I even went through a phase where I was using it in a sprayer bottle to clean all the mirrors and surfaces in the house. In the depths of winter, when the windows weren't open too often, I have to admit that it didn't smell great. Now I dilute it with lavender and tea tree oil and the smell is more pleasant. You'll be amazed at how effective it is.

RAW CACAO POWDER: Not to be confused with cocoa powder, raw cacao is unprocessed and very bitter, but it has a high nutritional content.

TAMARI: Tamari is a deeply savoury gluten-free soy sauce. You could of course use soy sauce instead, but I find soy sauce stronger so I would advise using half the amount initially and adding more if required.

SWEETENER: There is a lot of debate about honey in a vegan diet. Personally, I feel that as I'm aware of the need to support and maintain bee welfare, buying honey from eco-aware, organic, high-standard producers supports the important work they are doing and gives them an incentive to maintain their hives. Otherwise, agave syrup, maple syrup or coconut sugar are my preferred vegan sweeteners.

VEGAN VEGETABLE STOCK CUBES OR BOUILLON: I have included a recipe for homemade vegetable stock, but there are great vegan stock cubes, including some organic ones, on the market. Try a few and see which you prefer. Dissolving them in hot water before adding to soup adds an instant boost of flavour and seasoning. I prefer to use bouillon, which is loose grains, rather than a cube, as it's easier to adjust the quantities.

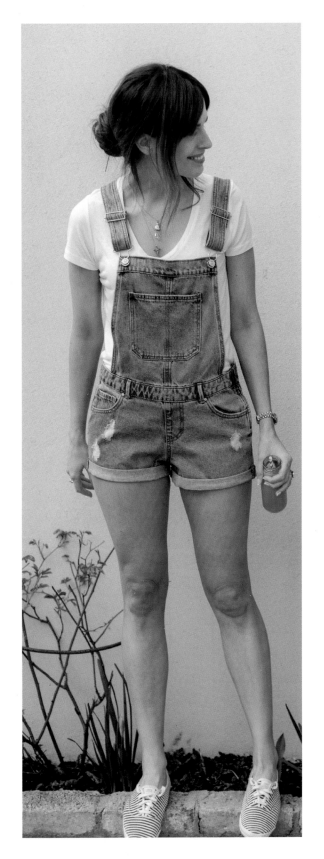

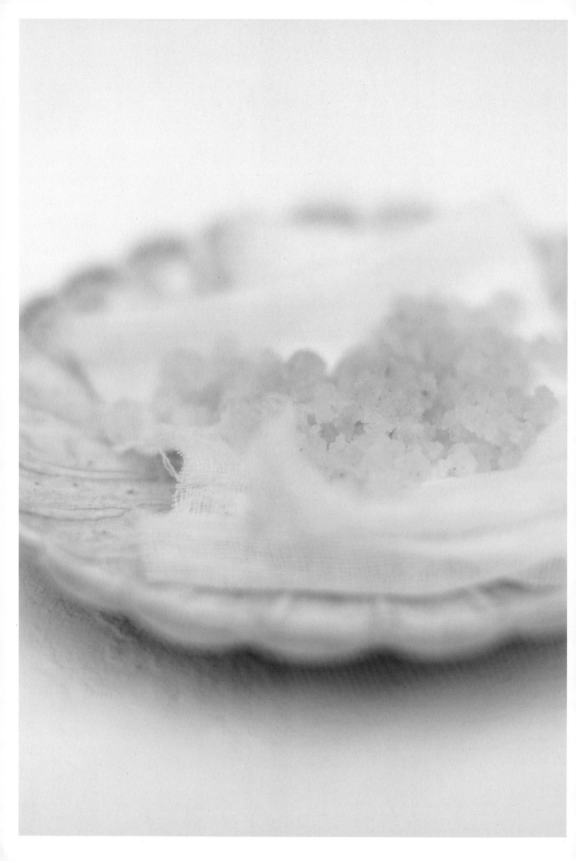

GET THE GEAR

The following are my suggestions for the tools to invest in to equip your kitchen. Thankfully, most vegan staples can now be easily found, so for example if you're contemplating buying a spiralizer, most supermarkets now sell packs of spiralized vegetables so you can try them a few times before taking the plunge. If you find yourself constantly buying energy balls, a good food processor will be a worthwhile purchase, and once you start making your own almond milk you'll be blown away by the taste compared to the shop-bought versions.

STRONG FOOD PROCESSOR

To make nut butters and energy balls, you really do need a high-powered food processor. Processing dates and grinding nuts puts a lot of pressure on a motor, so you need a strong wattage, otherwise it will soon burn out. Even with a strong machine it takes a solid 10 minutes for a nut butter to form the right consistency. The one I use has a 950 watt motor and came with a seven-year warranty. It also came with a price tag that put me into a state of shock for about an hour, but it has been put to the test for over three years now and has been a worthwhile investment.

HIGH-POWERED BLENDER

For making nut milks, smoothies, sauces and blending soups, a blender is essential. A high-powered blender has 1,000 to 1,560 watts of power and can do things that regular blenders can't. A high-powered blender liquefies leafy greens and vegetables in smoothies so that they go entirely unnoticed, blends soaked cashews to a mousse-like purée in moments and makes almond milk super fast. Some come with travel cups that are great for taking your morning smoothie with you and saving on washing up a separate cup.

COLD-PRESS JUICER

A cold-press juicer uses a low heat and grinds the fruit to a pulp, as opposed to a juicer with a fast-spinning metal blade that generates heat, which destroys some of the enzymes in the fruits and vegetables you're juicing. Since very little heat is used, the juice stays fresh for up to three days in the fridge, so you can make it in advance. It's a bit slower and more chopping is required, but it saves time in the long run as I usually make my juice the night before.

I rarely buy ready-made juice as I know that for the price of the vegetables, which is pretty nominal, I can make an amazing glass of fresh juice in a matter of minutes, so this has definitely been a good buy.

SPIRALIZER

I don't recommend the hand-operated versions, as I have seen and heard of too many accidents from using them. I have a horizontal spiralizer and all parts can be washed in the dishwasher. It's also very light and easy to store in the cupboard. For courgetti, carrot and squash noodles, a spiralizer is essential. At a push you could use a vegetable peeler instead, but it will be a lot more work.

DEHYDRATOR

I use my dehydrator for kale crisps and crackers and they can also be used for fermentation and tempering chocolate, but it isn't essential and they tend to take up a lot of kitchen counter real estate. I wouldn't consider it to be a high priority unless you're passionate about raw 'cooking', which is where ingredients are not heated above 116°F (47°C), thus keeping the nutrients intact while your food is dried and preserved.

HAND-HELD BLENDER

A hand-held blender saves you washing up a separate jug when blending soups and sauces, as you can use it directly in the pot. Most come with a whipping element, which is handy for mixing cake batters, again without a separate bowl to wash up.

AIRTIGHT CONTAINERS AND FLASKS

The best $10 you can spend is on some airtight containers in the dollar store. For meal prepping or eating on the go, sealable dishwasher- and freezer-safe airtight containers are a must. I try to avoid single-use plastics, so sandwich bags and the like are out and I look for reusable alternatives that I can wash easily.

If you want to have your soups and stews warm, a heated flask can keep them hot for up to 8 hours. Just make sure you temper the flask by pouring hot water in first to warm the barrel (or ice water if you want to keep something cold).

GOOD KNIVES

When I was growing up my dad was terrified of having sharp knives in the house, but interestingly I later discovered that most accidents occur because the knife isn't sharp enough. You'll be doing a lot of chopping, so a few good knives are essential. Investing in a small fruit knife is a good idea. They tend to be slightly rounded and are brilliant for removing the peel from citrus fruit. Most knives come with plastic casing that they can be stored in.

FRESH CHOPPING BOARDS

Some people have dedicated vegan kitchenware, i.e. pots and pans, but a chopping board that has never had meat on it is a nice fresh start. Try to get one in a different colour or one that's easily distinguishable from your existing boards. Make sure that those around you know that it's just for vegan food prep.

I also have a dedicated board for chopping onions and garlic, as I find that no matter how much you scrub, the smell lingers. It's only a small addition to your kitchen arsenal, but it stops desserts ever potentially having a lingering taste of onion!

Ensure there are child safety catches on all equipment. It amazes me that high-powered blenders can function at serious speed without the lid on. Avoid these.

Read the warranty and any conditions. Some warranties are voided if a part of the item is cleaned in the dishwasher, so double check this.

Wait for the deals! These are the kinds of item that are worth keeping an eye out for on Black Friday discount days. Try signing up for company newsletters for flash sales. They rarely go into the sale season, but there will often be special offers and once-off discounts.

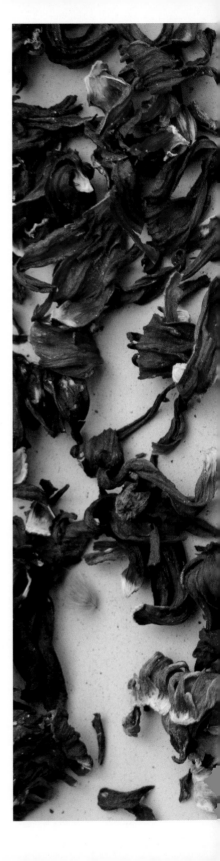

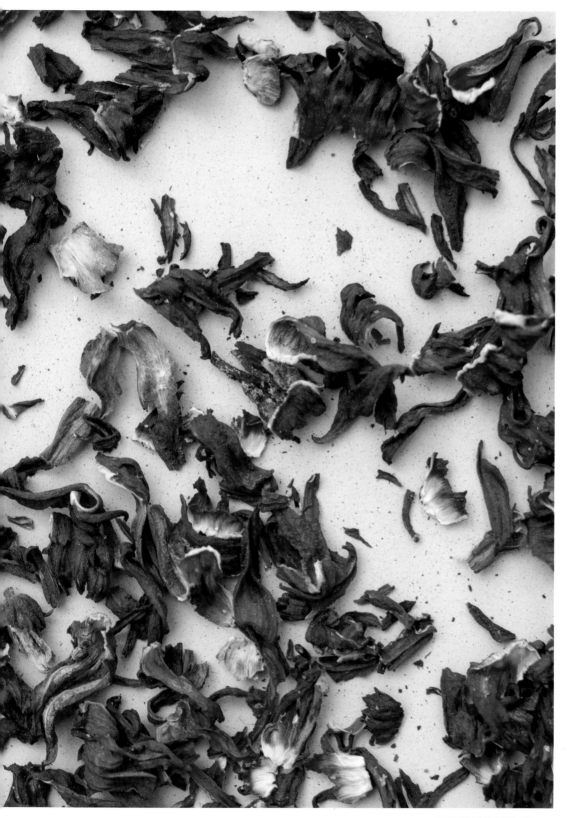

HELPFUL NOTES

HOW TO STERILISE JARS

There are no preservatives in any of the food I make, so good kitchen hygiene is essential. For storing nut butters, yogurts and chia jams or puddings, I always use jars fresh from the hottest wash in my dishwasher. If you have a baby bottle steriliser, that will do the job perfectly too.

You can also sterilise jam jars in the microwave, but not the mason jars that have metal clasps or any other kind of jar with metal on it. Clean the jars as normal with hot soapy water and rinse, but leave the jars a little wet. Microwave for 30–45 seconds, depending on the size of the jar. Let the jars cool for a few minutes before using or handling, as they could crack if you put them on a cold surface straight after heating them up.

Lids can be left in boiling water to sterilise. If you're using mason jars, remove the orange rubber seal and soak that in boiling water too.

Don't use old jam jar lids if they're damaged or rusty – they should be thrown away. Never use anything that's chipped or cracked.

SOAKING NUTS

A lot of recipes in this book call for soaking nuts before you use them. This is because nuts can be hard to digest on their own, but soaking them makes them easier to digest. If you are processing them, it also helps them to break down more easily. And in the case of cashews, they have an entirely different texture when soaked and blended.

A handy tip is that you can freeze nuts after they've been soaked and rinsed. This makes your morning smoothie or nut milk prep much quicker, plus freezing the nuts has the added advantage of making smoothies much creamier and it prevents your nut milk warming up during blending.

If you're stuck for time, you can also boil cashews for 15 minutes. The texture won't be as smooth as soaking, but it will help them blend. The recipes in this book refer to pre-soaked weight for all nuts.

NUT BUTTER SHELF LIFE

Unlike commercial nut butters, homemade versions don't contain preservatives that help to prevent bacterial growth, which eventually leads to spoilage. Although refrigeration doesn't kill bacteria, it does slow its growth. Packed in a tightly sealed container, nut butter keeps for up to one month in the fridge.

If you're gifting a jar of your homemade nut butter to someone, ensure you put a use-by label on the jar so that they can safely enjoy your thoughtful and delicious gift.

Homemade nut butter gets firmer after being in the fridge, which makes it harder to spread. Allow it to stand at room temperature for several minutes prior to serving. Immediately after use, reseal the jar tightly and pop it back in the fridge.

Juicing was a revelation for me. As strange as it sounds, I didn't like a lot of vegetables and fruit growing up, so coming up with ways to integrate them into juices really helped me explore different tastes. In terms of combinations, I would encourage you to get creative, and also go with what's practical and available. Whether you want something pure and green like Reset Juice, or something indulgent and chocolatey like Raw Chocolate Heaven, it's all in here.

JUICES & SMOOTHIES

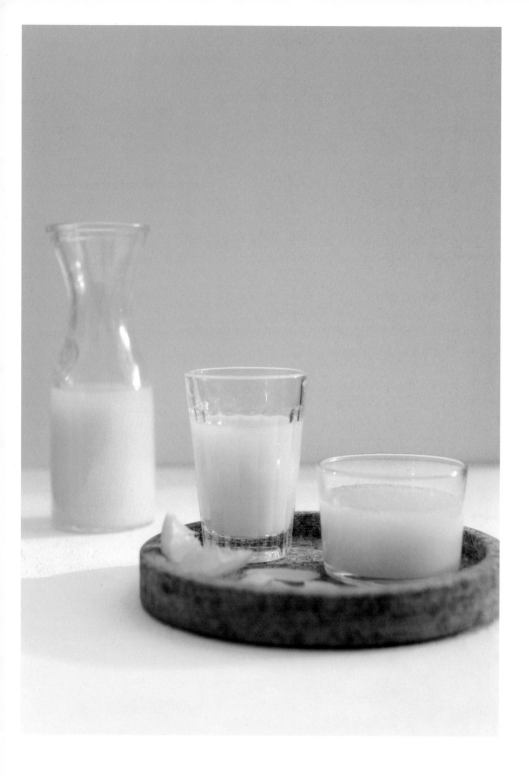

LEMON GINGERADE

1   Push the lemons and ginger through a juicer. I always follow it with approx. 3⅓ fl oz (100ml) of filtered water to wash all the juice through. Stir in the sweetener and dilute with the filtered or sparkling water. Serve ice cold.

2   You can keep the concentrate in a sealed bottle or jar for up to four days in the fridge.

This is pure refreshment on so many levels, plus all the warming powers of ginger. It's delicious on its own, but if you are so inclined, pouring it over a shot of vodka and lots of crushed ice is gorgeous too! You might need to add a little more sweetener – just stir in enough to suit your preference. I like to put the (peeled) lemons and ginger through my cold-press juicer as I get more juice out, but you could also use a hand-held citrus juicer and grate in the ginger if you don't have a juicer.

Makes 4¼ cup (1 litre)

6 lemons, peeled
1 x 2" (5cm) piece of peeled fresh
   ginger
6 tablespoons maple or agave syrup
4¼ cup (1 litre) filtered or sparkling
   water

RESET JUICE

During really busy phases of recipe testing or after a few indulgent days, I find myself craving greens and something simple. This juice does exactly what its name says – for me, it feels like a reset button. It's not sweet, is incredibly pure and is packed with vital greens.

You should always buy the best ingredients you can, but this is one time where I would advise trying to find organic cucumbers, as they are 95% water and make up a lot of this drink.

Makes 4¼ cups (1 litre)

2 cucumbers, preferably organic

2 celery stalks

1 apple

1 orange, peeled

1 lemon, peeled

1 x 1" (2.5cm) piece of fresh ginger

1 teaspoon super greens or spirulina
    powder (optional)

1 probiotic capsule, split open
    (optional)

1   Push all the ingredients through a juicer. I always follow it with approx. 3⅓ fl oz (100ml) of filtered water to wash all the juice through. Stir in the optional extras (if using). Use the back of a spoon to break up any clumps that form.

2   Using a cold-press juicer means that the juice will keep in the fridge for up to three days. I usually drink half and save the second half for the following day.

BEETROOT AND ORANGE QUENCH

1 Push all the ingredients through a juicer. I always follow it with 3⅓ fl oz (100ml) of filtered water to wash all the juice through. If you would like it to be sweeter, add another apple or orange or stir in some maple syrup.

TIP: To turn this into a thick, creamy smoothie, blend it with a few ice cubes, a banana and a tablespoon of chia seeds.

Fresh beetroot will ruin all your chopping boards and stain your hands for a few hours, but it's also earthy and rich, so all is forgiven. I just wash and scrub it well, then cut off the root. I like my juices quite sour, but by all means feel free to stir in a little maple syrup or liquid sweetener.

Serves 2

2 large carrots
1 apple
1 fresh beetroot, scrubbed well and
   root cut off
1 orange, peeled
1 lemon, peeled
1 x 1" (2.5cm) piece of fresh ginger

PINEAPPLE AND LEMON QUENCH

Sweet, refreshing and tangy, this really hits the spot when you want something sweet but healthy. Try to cut your pineapple skin off as close to the inner fruit as possible, as a lot of nutrients are just below the skin. Peel the citrus fruits and juice them whole, as there is so much more flavour to be found than just by using a citrus juicer.

Serves 2

2 apples
1 lemon, peeled
1 orange, peeled
½ large pineapple or 1 small one
1 x 2" (5cm) piece of fresh ginger

1   Press all the fruit through a juicer. I always follow it with 3⅓ fl oz (100ml) of filtered water to wash all the juice through. Serve over ice.

TIP: To make this creamy, stir in 1 tablespoon of coconut cream from a tin (see page 309).

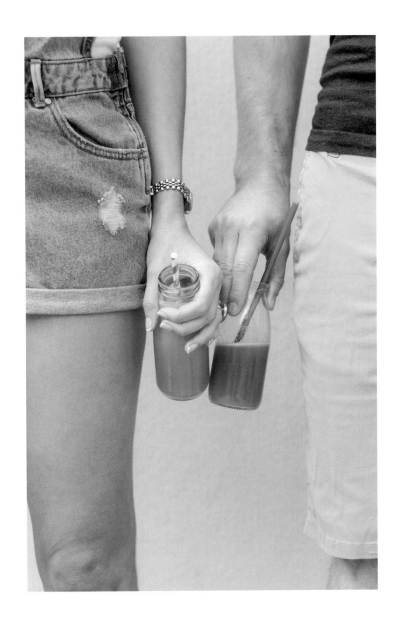

BITTER GREENS JUICE

Similar to the reset juice on page 36, this is as green as it gets. When I make juices I want as much dark leafy greens as possible in a short, sharp juice. If you're a fan of wheatgrass juice, you know that small juices can be powerful!

Serves 2

1 cucumber, preferably organic

1 celery stalk

1 large leaf of kale

1 lemon, peeled

1 teaspoon super greens or spirulina
    powder (optional)

1 probiotic capsule, split open
    (optional)

1   Push all the ingredients through a juicer. I always follow it with 3⅓ fl oz (100ml) of filtered water to wash all the juice through. If it's too bitter, add an apple, some pineapple or a little maple syrup, depending on how much more sweetness you need. Stir in the optional extras (if using).

TIP: Be careful not to overdo it with kale. The flavour is overpowering, so less is more. Even just a little too much can ruin a juice.

BERRY BOOST SMOOTHIE

1 Simply put all the ingredients except the almonds in a high-powered blender and blitz for approximately 30 seconds, until smooth. At this point I like to throw in a handful of almonds and pulse them for a few seconds, not enough to make them completely disappear, but just enough to give the smoothie some texture. Serve immediately or the chia seeds will make the smoothie too thick.

I usually have a smoothie for breakfast every day, as it can be put together and blitzed up in a matter of minutes and it really sets me up for the day. I work from home so I can pick from leftovers or make my own food during the day, but on days when I know I won't have as much control, I always make sure I have a good breakfast and sometimes that includes adding a boost of vegan protein powder to my smoothie, as I've done here. Trust me on the spinach – you won't notice the taste of it at all.

Serves 2

3½ oz (100g) frozen berries
1 banana
a handful of baby spinach
2 Medjool dates, pitted
1 scoop of vegan protein powder
    (optional)
1½ cup (350ml) almond milk
1 tablespoon chia seeds or flaxseeds
a small handful of almonds

RAW CHOCOLATE HEAVEN

If I had to pick a turning point in my opinion of vegan food, it would be shortly after I turned 27, when I was living in LA. Through a series of events that only make sense when you're a struggling actress who really should have gone home months ago, I found myself meeting a friend of an acupuncturist I had been to back in Dublin. Stella had lived in LA for over 20 years and is a raw vegan. At the time it was like another world I had no clue about. I couldn't even begin to imagine what her day-to-day diet might have looked like. She suggested we meet in Café Gratitude, which is a famous west coast vegan restaurant. The excellent documentary *May I Be Frank* centres on one of their eateries.

I perused the menu, not really sure what to order, when a raw chocolate smoothie caught my eye. When it arrived, I took one sip and something very strange and unexpected happened. It tasted rich, creamy, thick, chocolatey and like a total indulgence. Were we not in a place so virtuous, I would have assumed it was 'bad' for me. It tasted like heaven and I returned for it several times afterwards.

This smoothie piqued my interest in vegan cuisine and I've never turned back. This was the moment when I felt that food could be delicious as well as healthy – it essentially started the domino effect that led me to where I am now. I make my own version of it at home and I think you'll agree that it's gorgeous!

Serves 2

1 Put all the ingredients except the mint in a high-powered blender and blitz until smooth.

2 I have come to really like the bitterness of raw cacao, so I usually add a dusting of it to the top of a smoothie. If you prefer a sweeter flavour, a little drizzle of maple or agave syrup over the top looks and tastes gorgeous. Top with fresh mint (if using).

TIP: If you're using frozen avocado or banana, take them out of the freezer and allow to thaw for a few minutes while you prep your other ingredients, as they can be hard on the blades of your blender.

1 banana

½ ripe avocado, peeled and stoned

5 Medjool dates, pitted

1½ cup (350ml) plant milk

2 tablespoons raw cacao powder, plus extra for dusting

1 tablespoon lucuma powder (optional, but it makes it taste like caramel)

½ teaspoon vanilla extract

4 ice cubes (omit if using frozen avocado or banana)

maple or agave syrup, to sweeten (optional)

fresh mint, to garnish (optional)

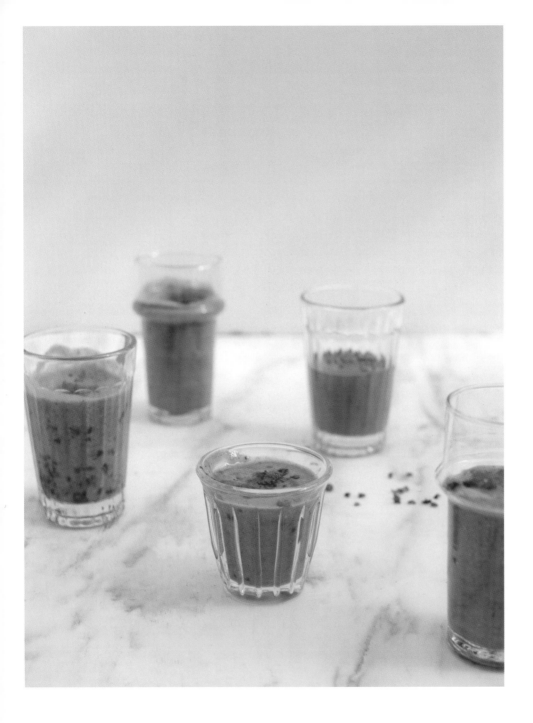

SUPER GREEN THICKSHAKE

1   Blitz all the ingredients in a high-powered blender until smooth. Make sure to use the plunger function to push the avocado down to give it a little help. If it's too thick add a little water to dilute it, but as the ice melts it will naturally thin it.

TIPS: If you're using frozen avocado or banana, take them out of the freezer and allow to thaw for a few minutes while you prep your other ingredients, as they can be hard on the blades of your blender. Likewise, if you don't have a high-powered blender, soak the dates in some hot water to soften them first.

Spirulina powder has to be blended into other foods as the taste is quite intense, but you won't notice it at all in this smoothie. Go for ½ teaspoon the first time you make it just to be sure you're happy with the taste.

Having both a juicer and a blender to clean in one go can seem a bit much, but if you use a cold-press juicer your green juice will stay fresh for three days in the fridge, so it can be made in advance.

A green juice is too small a breakfast for me, but by adding the avocado, banana and chia seeds plumps it up and it becomes filling and satisfying. It's deliciously creamy, packed full of super greens and will keep you full right up till lunch.

Serves 2

1 banana
½ ripe avocado, peeled and stoned
2 Medjool dates, pitted
1½ cup (350ml) reset juice (page 36)
1 heaped teaspoon spirulina powder
1 teaspoon chia seeds
a handful of ice

LIME AND COCONUT SHAKE

One day I had some leftover coconut milk after making an ambitiously large batch of coconut yogurt – more on that later. With a song dancing around my head I set out to create something with it that would work as a snack.

Initially I needed recipe guidelines for everything I was making but as my confidence grew it became more about playing around with flavours. What I now know for sure is that most things can be saved, so don't be afraid to get creative with ingredients – particularly if you have leftover fruit that's about to turn. Most of the time it will turn into an interesting creation. This is one of my favourite interesting creations.

Serves 2

2 limes
1 ripe avocado, peeled and stoned
1 banana, frozen
2 Medjool dates, pitted
approx. 1¼ cup (300ml) almond milk
1 teaspoon maca powder
ice cubes, to serve
1 tablespoon coconut milk (from a tin)
agave syrup, to sweeten (optional)

1   Zest one of the limes before juicing both of them, as doing it the other way around is much trickier! Add everything except the coconut milk and half of the zest to a high-powered blender and blitz until smooth.

2   Pour over ice, then swirl in the coconut milk and add the lime zest. If it's too sharp, swirl in a drizzle of agave syrup.

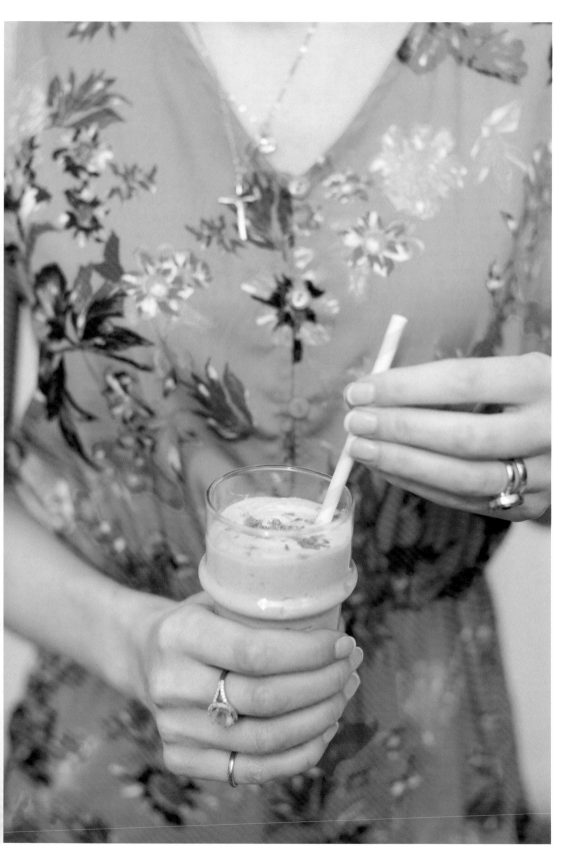

MOCHA AND HEMP SEED SHAKE

While I'm not one of those die-hard coffee addicts, I love a really good cup from time to time, plus sometimes you need that buzz. Whether it's been a sleepless night or you just want a lift, this is a delicious way to get it. You can of course use decaf coffee or leave it out completely if you like. Just add a little more cacao and know that it will be a more chocolatey shake.

Serves 2

2 tablespoons shelled hemp seeds

approx. 1¼ cup (300ml) almond milk

1 banana

3 Medjool dates, pitted

1–2 shots of espresso, depending on
    how much you need!

1 heaped tablespoon raw cacao
    powder

ice cubes, to serve

1   Put the hemp seeds in a high-powered blender with 3⅓ fl oz (100ml) of the almond milk and blitz for approximately 20 seconds to break down the seeds a bit. Add the rest of the ingredients and blend again until smooth. Serve over ice.

TIP: The hemp seeds make the smoothie creamy and also add texture. Feel free to use expresso powder if you don't have a coffee maker.

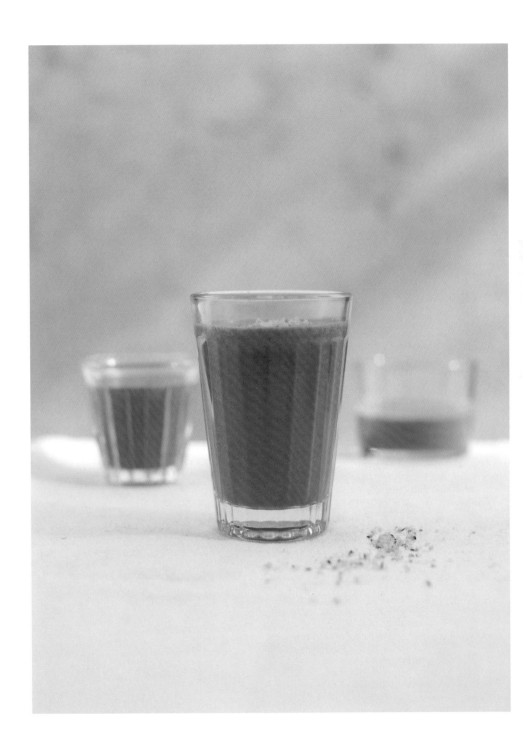

Breakfast is one of my favourite meals of the day. Vegan breakfast options can still be limited when eating out and it amazes me as there is so much potential. Whether you're looking for sweeter options like pancakes, granola and yogurt, or more savoury dishes like Turmeric Chickpea Scramble and Tamari Mushrooms, there are so many possibilities.

BREAKFAST

NATURAL COCONUT YOGURT WITH TINNED COCONUT MILK

Coconut yogurt is a staple in my diet and it really helped me to transition to this different way of eating. Initially I was buying it only a few times a month as a treat, as it can be quite expensive, but now I regularly make my own.

I make coconut yogurt with tinned coconut milk and also with fresh young coconut meat (see page 54), but this isn't as readily available. This recipe, though simple, requires the basics to be done precisely or else it won't work.

I've tried a lot of brands of coconut milk and found that brands do differ. The most important thing to look for, though, is that it's the full-fat milk, never the low-fat version, as it's the cream you want.

Serves 4

2 x approx. 1¾ cup (400ml) tins of full-fat coconut milk, preferably organic

1 tablespoon organic sugar or agave syrup, plus extra to taste

2 probiotic capsules, split open

lemon juice, to taste (optional)

½ teaspoon arrowroot powder (optional – see the tip opposite)

1 Put your two tins of coconut milk in the fridge for a few hours. This will cause the cream on top to harden, making it easier to separate the liquid.

2 Without shaking the tins, open them, then turn them upside down and drain out the water. Don't throw out the coconut water – save it for adding to smoothies or use it in the turmeric chickpea scramble (page 60), soups, casseroles or desserts.

3 Scoop out the thick cream and put it in a saucepan set on a very low heat. Gently warm it, then stir in the sugar or agave syrup. Don't allow it to boil – keep it on low heat. Remove the pan from the heat and gently stir in the split-open probiotic capsules.

4 Pour the mixture into a sterilised mason jar or jam jar. (See the note on page 30 on how to sterilise jars.) Put the jar in a warm, dark place away from draughts, with the lid slightly ajar and a muslin cloth or tea towel secured with an elastic band draped on top to stop any dust or flies getting in. A hot water tank/airing cupboard is perfect, or if you have a drawer or cupboard in your kitchen that is near the oven, the heat will help it develop. Leave it for 48 hours and you will see bubbles starting to form. This is the probiotic action taking place. During cooler months, I leave mine up to three days.

5 After 48 hours, taste it and feel free to add a little lemon juice or more sweetener depending on whether you like it more tart or sweet.

6 If you want the yogurt to thicken up a bit more, gently stir in the arrowroot powder, then transfer to the fridge, where it will keep for up to a week. The cold fridge will also help to set the yogurt.

TIPS: As there are no stabilisers or thickeners in this yogurt, it can be quite runny. Ensuring you use only the creamiest coconut milk helps combat this. Adding the arrowroot powder will help to thicken it a little.

Don't clean the jar if you're making a new batch of yogurt straightaway. Just add it into the same jar and some of the good bacteria will act as an extra starter for your next batch of yogurt.

NATURAL COCONUT YOGURT WITH FRESH YOUNG COCONUT MEAT

On the first day I visited Thailand, I discovered fresh young coconuts, which are cut open right in front of you. Every day after that was punctuated by finding one.

Coconuts are easily accessible and cheap in Thailand, ranging from 40 Baht (approx. $1) on the street to 100 Baht (approx. $2.75) in hotels and restaurants, but you'd be surprised how often you can find them here. I pick them up in the Asia Market in Dublin.

Before you try to chop open your coconuts, go online and watch several videos of how to do it first. It's not difficult, but a sharp, heavy knife and quite a bit of force are required. Once they're opened, you can easily drain the water and scoop out the flesh with a metal spoon.

Serves 4

2 fresh young coconuts (approx. 3½ oz [100g] flesh)

1 cup (250ml) coconut water

1 tablespoon organic sugar or agave syrup, plus extra to taste

2 probiotic capsules, split open

lemon juice, to taste (optional)

1 Crack open the coconuts, making sure you save the water. Add the coconut flesh and about one-quarter of the coconut water to a blender and blitz until it's broken down to a creamy paste. Add the remaining coconut water and blend again. You want it to be thick, so don't add too much water. Add the sugar and probiotics and pulse the blender lightly to disperse.

2 Pour the mixture into a sterilised mason jar or jam jar. (See the note on page 30 on how to sterilise jars.) Put the jar in a warm, dark place away from draughts, with the lid slightly ajar and a muslin cloth or tea towel secured with an elastic band draped on top to stop any dust or flies from getting in. A hot water tank cupboard/airing cupboard is perfect, or if you have a drawer or cupboard in your kitchen that is near the oven, the heat will help it develop. Leave it for 48 hours and you will see bubbles starting to form. This is the probiotic action taking place. During cooler months, I leave mine up to three days.

3 After 48 hours, taste it and feel free to add a little lemon juice or more sweetener depending on whether you like it more tart or sweet.

4 Transfer to the fridge, where it will keep for up to a week.

TIPS: Some recipes say not to add any sugar, but I find it gives the probiotics a kick-start. Don't use honey, as it's a natural antibacterial agent and will therefore kill the live bacteria that you need to activate the yogurt.

Don't clean the jar if you're making a new batch of yogurt straightaway. Just add it into the same jar and some of the good bacteria will act as an extra starter for your next batch of yogurt.

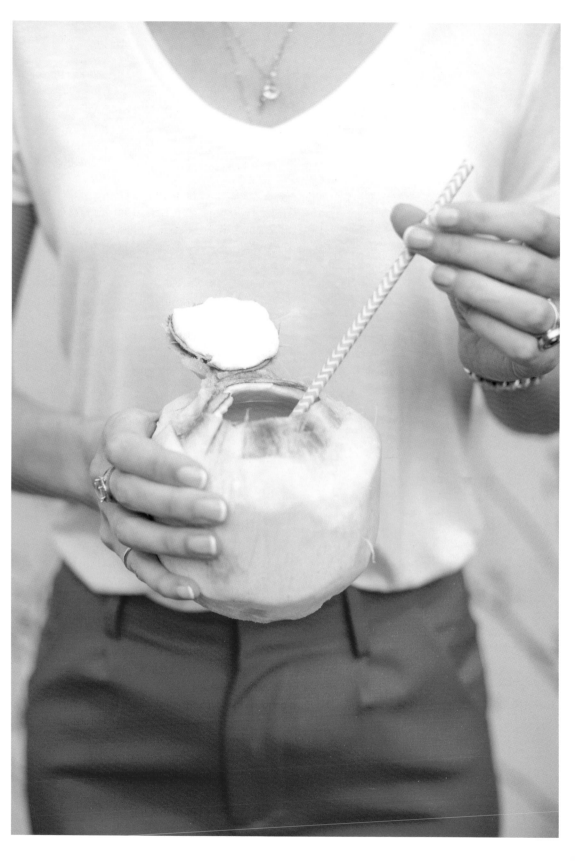

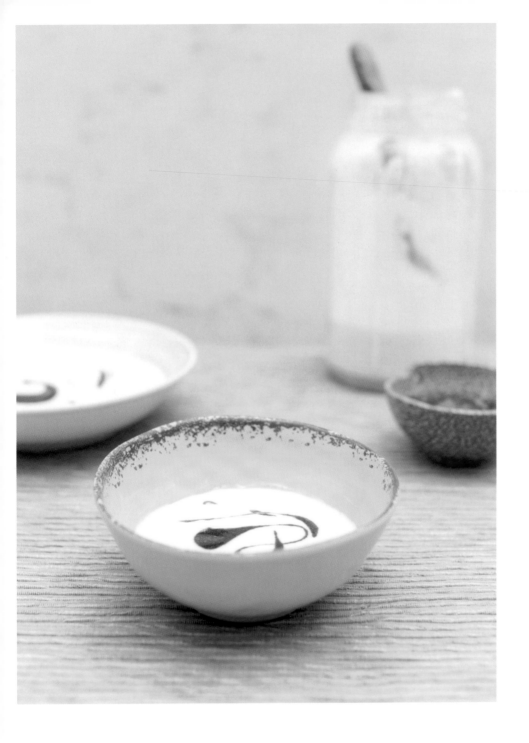

VANILLA COCONUT YOGURT WITH RASPBERRIES

1   Put the berries and water in a saucepan and simmer until softened. If you're using frozen berries, it should take approximately 8 minutes to defrost and soften them. Stir in the vanilla, maple or agave syrup and the lemon juice.

2   Remove the pan from the heat and allow the mixture to cool. Ensure most of the liquid has evaporated before you fold it into your yogurt or it will make it too runny. You can either give it a beautiful raspberry ripple effect or you can mix it in thoroughly.

3   To serve, top with berries and a further drizzle of maple or agave syrup. Store covered in the fridge for up to a week.

I love yogurt that's so tart that it almost makes you wince, but I'm well aware that it's not for everyone! This vanilla and raspberry yogurt is so beautiful and makes an ideal centrepiece if you're having people around for a lazy brunch.

Serves 4

3½ oz (100g) fresh or frozen raspberries or mixed berries, plus extra to serve

2 tablespoons filtered water

2 vanilla pods, cut in half lengthways and seeds scraped out

1 tablespoon maple or agave syrup

2 teaspoons lemon juice

1 batch of coconut yogurt (see page 52 or page 54)

CASHEW YOGURT WITH A BLUEBERRY SWIRL

Deliciously rich and creamy cashew yogurts are easy to make, and you can also control the thickness.

Serves 4

7 oz (200g) cashew nuts

a pinch of sea salt or Himalayan
　　pink salt

6¾ fl oz (200ml) filtered or cooled
　　boiled water or kefir (page 264)

1 tablespoon raw cane organic sugar
　　or agave syrup

2 probiotic capsules, split open

FOR THE BLUEBERRY SWIRL:

3 oz (80g) fresh or frozen blueberries

2 tablespoons filtered water

1 tablespoon agave syrup or other
　　sweetener (optional)

2 teaspoons lemon juice (optional)

1　Put the cashews in a bowl with a pinch of sea salt or Himalayan pink salt, cover with filtered water and soak for at least 8 hours or ideally overnight, then drain and rinse. (See the note on page 30 on soaking nuts.)

2　Put the cashews in a blender with ¼ cup (50ml) of the water or kefir and blend thoroughly. Add a little more water if the mixture isn't gelling, but you want to keep it concentrated at the early stages so it gets really smooth. Once it's smooth, drizzle in enough of the remaining water or kefir until your desired consistency is achieved. Pulse in the sugar or agave syrup, then stir in the probiotics at the last moment.

3　You can eat this immediately or you can allow the good bacteria to multiply by transferring the yogurt to a sterilised mason jar or jam jar. (See the note on page 30 on how to sterilise jars.) Put the jar in a warm, dark place away from draughts, with the lid slightly ajar and a muslin cloth or tea towel secured with an elastic band draped on top to stop any dust or flies getting in. A hot water tank cupboard/airing cupboard is perfect, or if you have a drawer or cupboard in your kitchen that is near the oven, the heat will help it to develop. Leave it for 48 hours and you will see bubbles starting to form. This is the probiotic action taking place.

4　Whether you'll be eating the yogurt straight away or allowing it to ferment, put it in the fridge to set for at least 3 hours before serving.

5   To make the blueberry swirl, simmer the berries in the water until a thick compote has formed. Mash the berries to a purée with the back of a fork. Remove the pan from the heat and allow the mixture to cool. Stir in the sweetener if required, or if you prefer it more tart, omit the sweetener altogether. You can add a squeeze of fresh lemon juice if you would like it to be more sharp.

6   Ensure most of the liquid has evaporated before you fold the blueberries into your yogurt or it will make it too runny. You can either give it a beautiful ripple effect or you can mix it in thoroughly. Store in a sealed jar in the fridge for up to five days.

TIP: You need a sterile environment for your ferment to thrive, so always use filtered water. If you're unsure, boil some water in the kettle and allow it to cool before using.

TURMERIC CHICKPEA SCRAMBLE

I discovered Chickpea Scramble one lazy Sunday morning. Craving something satisfying and savory for breakfast I experimented with chickpeas and wondered why it had taken me so long. This is satisfying, quick and tasty. Enjoy!

Serves 2

olive oil, for frying and to serve

2 shallots, finely chopped

1 x 14 oz (400g) tin of chickpeas,
     drained and rinsed

1 tablespoon boiling water

1 garlic clove, crushed

1 tablespoon nutritional yeast

1 tablespoon coconut cream from a
     tin (see page 308) or 2 tablespoons
     leftover coconut water

½ teaspoon ground turmeric

½ teaspoon garlic powder

¼ teaspoon black salt

freshly ground black pepper

tamari mushrooms (page 61),
     to serve

garlicky sautéed kale (page 154),
     to serve

1 ripe avocado, peeled, stoned
     and sliced, to serve

1   Heat a splash of olive oil in a frying pan set over a medium heat. Add the shallots and lightly fry for about 5 minutes, until transparent.

2   While the shallots are cooking, put the chickpeas in a mixing bowl. Pour over the boiling water and mash them a little using the back of a fork or a potato masher. Add the crushed garlic, nutritional yeast, coconut cream, turmeric, garlic power and black salt. Mash everything together if you want a smoother consistency, but I think it's nice to leave a bit of texture.

3   Add the chickpeas to the pan with the shallots. Cook for a few minutes, stirring to ensure everything cooks evenly. If you want to mash it a bit more, go in with the potato masher and mash until it's your desired consistency. Add a drizzle of olive oil and salt and pepper to taste. Serve on warmed plates with the tamari mushrooms, garlicky kale and sliced avocado.

TIP: A full fry-up can be a one-pan affair. I usually make the scramble last, after the mushrooms and kale have been cooked and are staying warm in the oven, so there's no need to wash the pan in between. The flavours are all similar and if anything actually enhance the taste, plus it saves on washing up.

Save the water from the tin of chickpeas for making the vegan meringues on page 208.

TAMARI MUSHROOMS

1   Heat a drizzle of olive oil in a frying pan set over a medium-high heat. Add the mushrooms and garlic and cook, stirring gently to ensure the garlic doesn't burn, for about 4 minutes. When the mushrooms start to soften, reduce the heat and add the tamari and thyme (if using). Stir to coat evenly and allow to cook for a further minute.

2   Transfer to a hot plate to keep warm while you prep your other breakfast additions or enjoy immediately. Store any leftovers in an airtight container in the fridge for up to three days.

TIP: If you're going to be having these mushrooms on toast by themselves, you can make them a little creamier by adding a tablespoon of coconut milk and cooking for an extra minute. Pile them high onto sourdough toast spread with mashed avocado, a drizzle of olive oil and a bit of pepper. Tamari is naturally very savoury, so taste it before adding any salt.

Breakfast gets elevated to something special when these tamari mushrooms are involved. That said, they don't need to be reserved for weekends, as they can be cooked in under 5 minutes. This works well with all kinds of mushrooms if you happen to find lovely oyster mushrooms or more unusual kinds, but simple button mushrooms are fine too. As pack sizes vary, a general rule of thumb is to allow 3½ oz (100g) of mushrooms per person. I usually cook 7 oz (200g), even if it's just for myself, as any leftovers are handy to have in the fridge to liven up a simple salad or 10-minute meal.
Serves 2

olive oil, for frying

7 oz (200g) mushrooms, wiped clean
   and thinly sliced

2 garlic cloves, crushed

1 tablespoon tamari, soy sauce or
   coconut aminos

½ teaspoon finely chopped fresh
   thyme (optional)

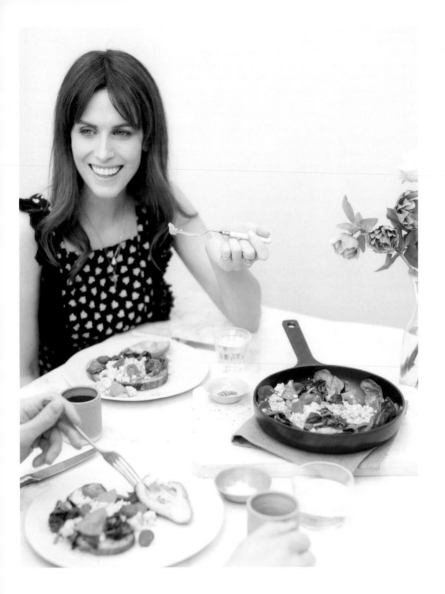

TIP: If you really want that eggy taste, black salt is a must. It may also be called kala namak and is sourced from northern India. It can be easily bought online and in most health food stores. It has a high sulphur content, which is what gives this dish a convincingly eggy flavour.

TOMATO TOFU SCRAMBLE WITH GARLIC SPINACH

1   Preheat the oven to 175°F (80°C) and put a serving plate in it to warm.

2   Remove the tofu from the package and pat it dry with kitchen paper to remove as much of the water as possible. Crumble the tofu into a bowl, then add the milk, turmeric, onion powder and a pinch of black salt and pepper and mash to combine.

3   Drizzle some olive oil in a frying pan set over a medium heat. Add the garlic and lightly fry for about 30 seconds before adding the spinach. Quickly toss the leaves to ensure they are coated in the garlic and oil. Once they're starting to wilt, remove the pan from the heat. Transfer the spinach to the warmed serving plate and keep warm in the oven.

4   Without washing the pan, add a little more oil if needed. Add the shallots and lightly sauté for a minute, then add the chopped tomato. When the shallots and garlic start to go golden, push everything to the side of the pan, then add the mashed tofu. Leave to heat through for a moment before stirring to ensure it cooks evenly. Mix in the tomatoes and garlic from the side of the pan, stirring to combine. Within 8 minutes, your tofu will be cooked and the shallots should have started to crisp. You can return the spinach to the pan to combine the two together or serve them separately if you like.

5   Transfer to warmed plates and top with a drizzle of oil and a pinch of chilli flakes (if using), then season to taste with extra salt and pepper. This goes really well with some sliced avocado or sourdough toast on the side.

Tofu is a blank canvas for flavours, but it needs to be properly prepped and seasoned to make it tasty. Whenever people tell me they don't like tofu, I want to cook this scramble for them. It so closely resembles scrambled eggs that it's hard to believe it's not the real thing.

Serves 4

1 x 14 oz (400g) block of firm tofu

splash of unsweetened plant-based milk

1 teaspoon ground turmeric

½ teaspoon onion powder

a pinch of black salt (see the tip below)

a pinch of freshly ground black pepper

olive oil, for frying

2 garlic cloves, crushed

a handful of baby spinach

2 shallots, finely chopped

1 ripe tomato or 4 cherry tomatoes, finely chopped

a pinch of chilli flakes (optional)

1 ripe avocado, peeled, stoned and sliced, to serve (optional)

sourdough toast, to serve (optional)

CREAMY GARLIC MUSHROOMS AND AVOCADO ON TOAST

Backstage at *The Six O'Clock Show* before my first appearance, one of the presenters was intrigued by my vegan lifestyle. What did I actually eat? Did I miss a Sunday fry-up? It had been years since I'd eaten, much less missed, a traditional fry-up as there are so many gorgeous options that are filling, satisfying and, most important, delicious. I went through my breakfast options, and when I described this one, his eyes lit up. 'That sounds like something I could really enjoy'.

This is ideal for a weekend brunch when there's a little more time to enjoy it. Grilled tomatoes make this an even more filling veggie breakfast. Add a fresh pot of tea and the papers for best effect!

Serves 2

2 ripe avocados, peeled and stoned

1 tablespoon raw apple cider vinegar
   or lemon juice

¼ teaspoon paprika (optional)

sea salt and freshly ground black
   pepper

olive oil, for frying

2 garlic cloves, crushed

7 oz (200g) mushrooms, chopped

½ teaspoon dried oregano

½ teaspoon dried sage

¾ cup (175ml) coconut milk (from a
   tin)

4 slices of bread, toasted

chopped fresh flat-leaf parsley, to
   garnish

1   Put the avocados, vinegar or lemon juice, paprika (if using) and some salt and pepper in a bowl and mash together with a fork.

2   Heat a splash of olive oil in a frying pan set over a medium-high heat. Add the garlic and lightly fry for 30 seconds, then add the mushrooms and sauté for 8 minutes, until softened. Stir in the oregano and sage and cook for a further minute to release the flavours. Add the coconut milk and simmer for 2 minutes.

3   Spread the toast with the mashed avocado, top with the piping-hot mushrooms and garnish with the chopped fresh parsley. Serve immediately on warmed plates.

TIPS: You can use your favourite bread here, but sourdough is particularly good as it stays firm even after all the toppings have been added.

The mushrooms are best served piping hot but they cook quickly, so if you're making this for a group, do your prep in advance and cook everything at the last minute.

Frozen avocados are now readily available, and while they work well in smoothies, they don't work here. Buying perfectly ripe avocados is a tricky business, but a simple trick is to remove the seed at the top and look at the colour of the flesh inside. If it's brown, put it down!

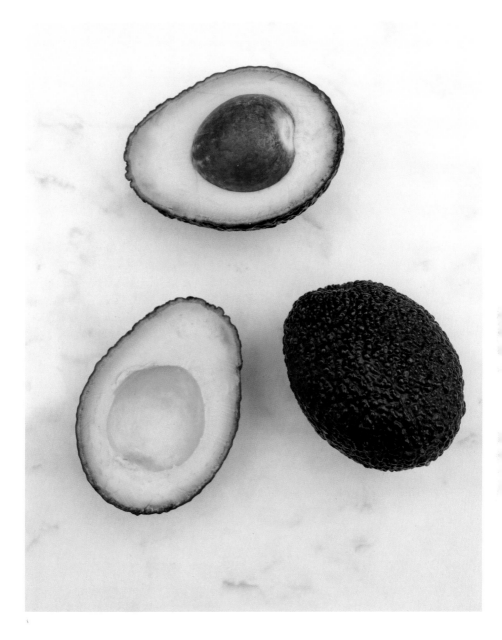

CANNELLINI BEANS IN TOMATO SAUCE

Pulses were a mystery to me a few years ago. It was an area, and an aisle of the supermarket, that I completely avoided, but pulses are an essential part of a plant-based diet. For this recipe I used tinned beans, which are readily available and quick to prepare, but feel free to substitute dried beans that you've soaked and boiled.

Serves 2

olive oil, for frying

2 onions, thinly sliced

1 garlic clove, minced

1 x 14 oz (400g) tin of cannellini
   beans, drained and rinsed

1 fresh red chilli, deseeded and
   finely chopped (optional)

½ teaspoon cumin seeds

1 cup (250ml) tomato passata

1 tablespoon tahini

sea salt and freshly ground
   black pepper

1 Heat a splash of olive oil in a frying pan set over a high heat. Add the onions and garlic and lightly fry for about 5 minutes, until the onions become translucent. Add the beans, chilli (if using) and cumin seeds, stirring to blend the flavours.

2 Add the passata, reduce the heat to medium and partially cover the pan with a lid. Simmer for 10 minutes, until most of the liquid has evaporated and you have a thick bean stew. Add the tahini and season to taste with salt and pepper. Leave to simmer with the lid off for 2–3 more minutes to reduce it down even more.

3 Serve in warmed shallow bowls with thick slices of toast and avocado or with a bowl of brown rice and some hummus.

TIP: This is also just as nice cold, so it works well as a protein-packed lunchbox option.

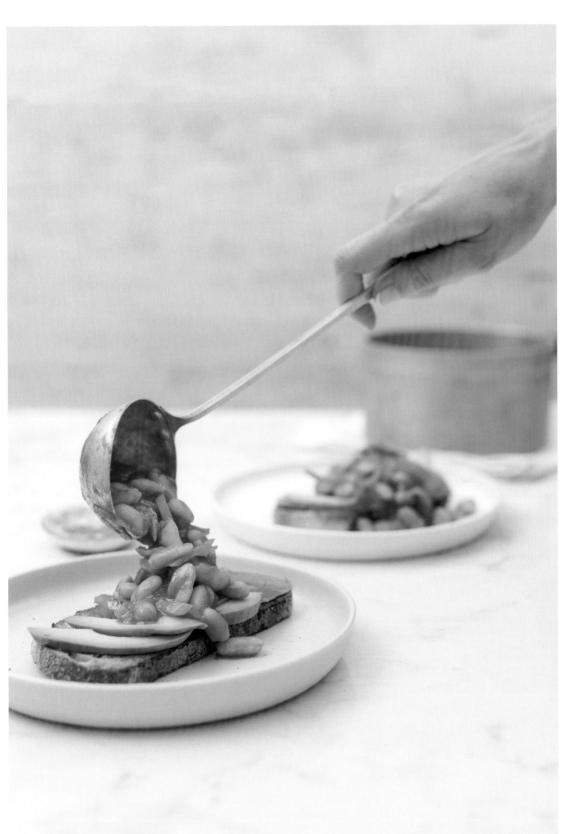

GRAIN-FREE BLUEBERRY AND QUINOA GRANOLA

Quinoa flakes have a really nutty flavour and are the perfect option for people who don't like oats. The crunchy, chewy texture of this granola is a really nice addition to the top of a smoothie or even just some simple natural yogurt. This is too expensive to eat by the bowlful, so I use it more as a topping. It's quite a sweet treat, but if you want to reduce the sweetness, simply omit the dates as there is enough natural sweetness from the maple or agave syrup and the blueberries.

Makes 16 small servings

3½ oz (100g) quinoa pops or flakes

3½ oz (100g) flaked coconut

1¾ oz (50g) chopped or flaked almonds

1½ oz (40g) pumpkin seeds

1 oz (30g) ground flaxseeds or chia seeds

½ teaspoon vanilla powder

½ teaspoon ground cinnamon

½ teaspoon fine sea salt

3 tablespoons coconut oil

2 tablespoons maple or agave syrup

1¾ oz (50g) dried blueberries

5 Medjool dates, pitted and finely chopped

1 tablespoon hemp seeds

1 Preheat the oven to 300°F (150°C). Line a baking tray or casserole dish with non-stick baking paper or foil.

2 Put the quinoa and half of the coconut flakes in a large bowl along with the almonds, seeds, vanilla, cinnamon and salt and mix together.

3 Melt the coconut oil and maple or agave syrup together in a small saucepan set over a low heat, then pour it over the dry ingredients, stirring until everything is evenly coated.

4 Transfer to the lined baking tray or dish and spread it out in an even layer. Bake in the oven for 15–20 minutes, stirring it once halfway through the cooking time to ensure that nothing is burning.

5 When the granola looks lightly toasted, remove it from the oven. While still warm, stir in the blueberries and dates.

6 I like the granola to clump up a bit, but if you prefer it to be more even, break up any big pieces with your hands and allow to cool. When it has cooled completely, stir in the remaining coconut flakes and the hemp seeds.

7 I keep this in an airtight container in the fridge, as I think it keeps it extra fresh, but it will also keep at room temperature for up to two weeks. If it goes a little too soft, heat it up in the oven for a few minutes to crisp it up again.

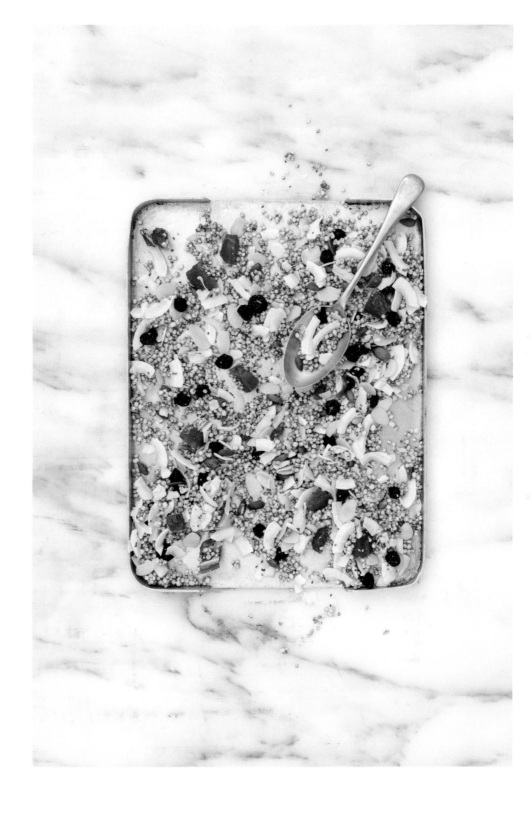

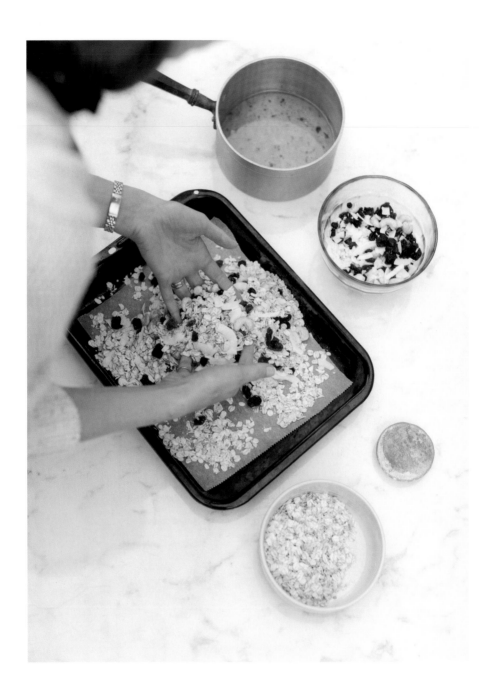

VANILLA AND COCONUT GRANOLA

When I was growing up, my mum made granola every week. She called it grits, which I now know is something totally different (it's a savoury, creamy corn porridge). She used to eat little saucers of it and you could almost locate her by following the trail of oats and seeds, which would likely lead to the phone or the conservatory, where she tended to her beloved plants.

There are a lot of granolas on the market, and while they all have their merits, nothing will ever beat what you make at home. This is pure comfort, and given that oats are incredibly cheap, especially if you bulk buy, it's a great way of economically feeding hungry families at breakfast. Plus, once you start making this regularly, you'll likely have a cupboard full of dried fruit and seeds and can personalise the recipe according to what you like or what you have available at the time.

Makes 12 servings

(continued)

14 oz (400g) rolled oats

2 oz (50g) buckwheat groats

2 oz (50g) desiccated coconut

1 teaspoon ground cinnamon

a pinch of sea salt

2 tablespoons melted coconut oil

4 tablespoons maple or agave syrup

1 teaspoon vanilla powder or 2 vanilla pods, cut in half lengthways and seeds scraped out (keep the pods)

approx. 3⅓ fl oz (100ml) filtered water

2 oz (50g) cashew nuts, lightly crushed

2 oz (50g) dried fruit, such as cranberries, blueberries, goji berries, raisins or chopped apricots

2 oz (50g) coconut flakes (if you can't find them, add an additional 1¾ oz (50g) desiccated coconut)

1   Preheat the oven to 400°F (200°C). Line as wide a baking tray as possible with non-stick baking paper or tin foil.

2   Put the oats, buckwheat, desiccated coconut, cinnamon and salt in a large bowl and mix together.

3   Melt the coconut oil in a little pan set over a low heat, then stir in the maple or agave syrup and the vanilla powder or seeds. If you use vanilla pods, add the scraped-out pods to the pan and keep it warm for up to 10 minutes to release every ounce of flavour. Remove the pods and set them aside, then stir in the water.

4   Pour the syrup over the dry ingredients and stir well to combine. Transfer to the lined tray in a single layer and bury the vanilla pods into the mix. I like it when it clumps up a bit, but if you want a more even texture, break up any clumps before placing the tray in the oven.

5   Bake in the oven for about 25 minutes. Check it halfway through to stir and turn the baking tray around to ensure it's not burning on one side. Remove the tray from the oven when there is a hint of golden brown appearing, as it will still continue to cook a bit. Remove the pods and discard them.

6   Immediately stir in the cashew nuts, dried fruit and coconut flakes (if using) while the granola is still warm. Allow to cool completely before transferring to a large mason jar. This will last for up to a fortnight, but if it goes a little soft, put your required portion into a warm oven for 6–8 minutes to crisp it up again.

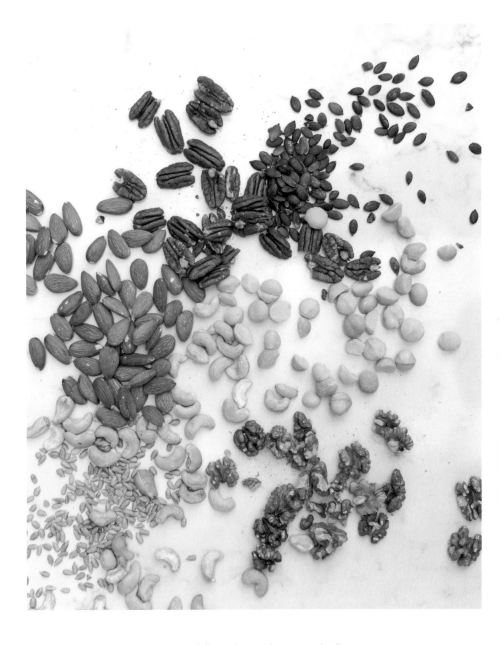

TIP: There are a few simple rules to follow when making granola. First, use the best-quality jumbo oats you can get, ideally organic. Porridge oats are fine, but you'll get a 'dusty' granola. Most combinations of nuts, seeds and dried fruit work, so don't worry if you don't have a particular ingredient. And always add dried fruit after the granola comes out of the oven, as it will quickly burn if you bake it. Stir it in when your granola is fresh out of the oven, while there is still enough heat to release the flavours from the fruit.

OAT AND CRANBERRY BREAKFAST BARS

The problem with making a batch of these and then assuming that your breakfast is now sorted for the week is that they tend to be enjoyed throughout the day or mysteriously disappear when other members of your household realise how tasty they are.

Makes 10 bars

5¼ oz (150g) cashew nuts

1¾ oz (50g) desiccated coconut or
   coconut flakes

3½ oz (100g) Medjool dates, pitted

1 banana, chopped

3½ oz (100g) rolled oats

1 tablespoon melted coconut oil or
   light vegetable oil

1 teaspoon maca powder

1¾ oz (50g) dried cranberries

1   Preheat the oven to 285°F (140°C). Grease a approx. 6" x 8" (15cm x 20cm) baking dish and line with non-stick baking paper.

2   Blitz the cashews in a food processor for about 15 seconds, until they are all broken down. Add the desiccated coconut or coconut flakes and pulse to combine, then add the dates a few at a time and blend well.

3   Add the banana, oats, coconut oil and maca powder and blend again until a thick paste forms. Add the cranberries and pulse briefly for about 10 seconds max.

4   Press the mixture into the prepared tin, then bake in the oven for 15 minutes.

5   Allow to cool and fully set before slicing into bars. You can store these in an airtight container in the fridge for up to a week, but I like them straight from the freezer, so see which way you like best.

TIPS: These bars can also be eaten raw, in which case you need to refrigerate them for 20 minutes to allow the coconut oil to set and the bars to firm up.

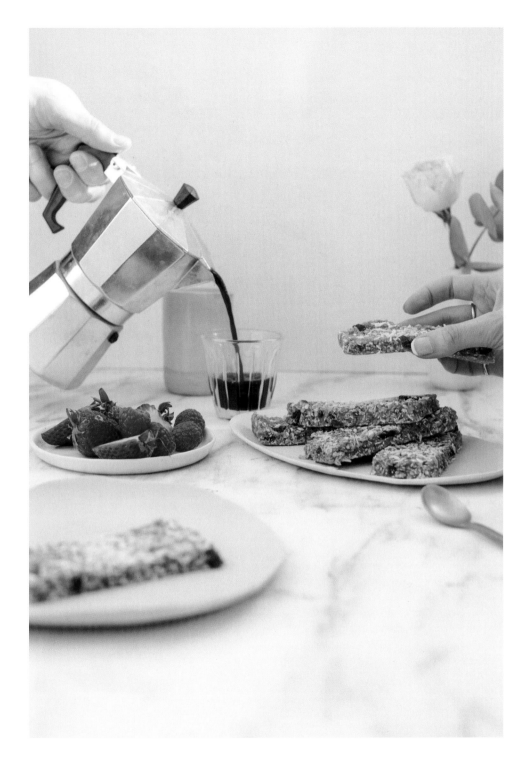

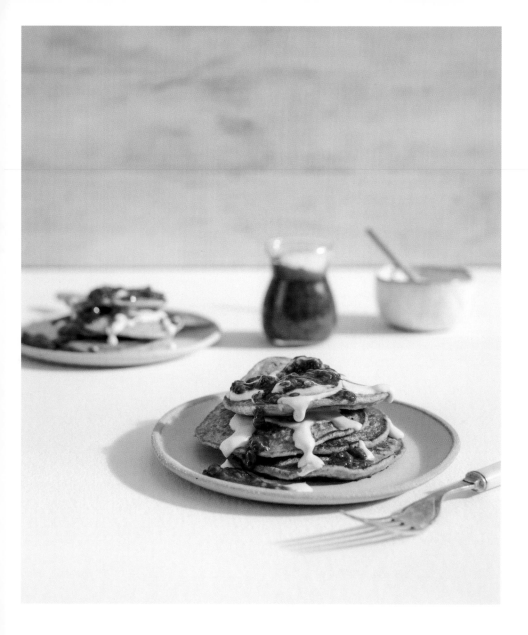

TIPS: The pancake batter will keep in the fridge overnight if you don't use it all or if you want to make it ahead of time. If you don't have spelt flour, you can blitz rolled oats in a food processor until they're a fine powder and use that instead. I use frozen mixed berries, but you can of course use fresh berries or just one type of berry if you like.

BERRY AND COCONUT CREAM PANCAKES

1 Preheat the oven to 175°F (80°C).

2 To make the pancake batter, simply put all the ingredients except the coconut oil in a blender and blitz to combine. It's best if you can leave it to rest for 10 minutes or so. Use this time to make the berry compote, put the plates in the oven to warm and brew the coffee.

3 To make the berry compote, put the berries and water in a small saucepan set over a medium heat and simmer for 10 minutes. When the berries are starting to soften, add the chia seeds, lemon juice and agave syrup. Remove from the heat and allow to cool for 10 minutes. Use a hand-held blender or pour it into a NutriBullet and blend to a creamy consistency.

4 Have a plate warming up in the oven to put your pancakes on as they cook to keep them hot.

5 Melt a little coconut oil in a hot pan, then pour a tablespoon of the pancake batter into the centre of the pan. You want each pancake to be about 4" (10cm) in diameter, so tilt the pan slightly to ensure the batter spreads evenly across the base. Cook for 1 minute, until bubbles start to form on the surface. Flip the pancake over and cook until the bottom is golden brown. Transfer to the hot plate in the oven to keep warm while you cook the rest of the pancakes.

6 To serve, stack up the pancakes on warmed plates, alternating with a layer of the berry compote and the vanilla coconut cream. Top with fresh berries and drizzle with maple syrup if you want a little extra sweetness.

I avoided pancakes for a while after a disastrous and expensive Pancake Tuesday when I tried several recipes and only ended up with a crumbly, greasy mess. These are gorgeous, but it's the toppings that make them special. The combination of the coconut cream and the sharp berries is heavenly, but you could go for something simpler like maple syrup and lemon as well.

Makes 12

6⅓ oz (180g) spelt flour or ground
  rolled oats (see the tip opposite)
1 banana
1 x approx. 1¾ cup (400ml) tin of
  coconut milk
4 tablespoons maple syrup
1 tablespoon chia seeds or flaxseeds
1 teaspoon baking powder or
  arrowroot powder
¼ teaspoon vanilla extract
coconut oil, for cooking

FOR THE BERRY COMPOTE:
3½ oz (100g) frozen mixed berries
4¼ fl oz (125ml) filtered water
1 tablespoon chia seeds
1 tablespoon lemon juice
1 tablespoon agave syrup

TO SERVE:
1 batch of vanilla coconut cream
  (page 309)
fresh berries
maple syrup

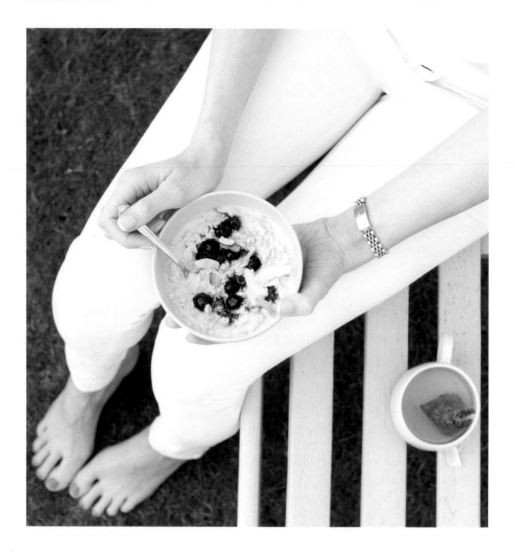

TIPS: When it comes to oats for porridge, I really don't like 'porridge' oats. I prefer the texture of jumbo oats and the overnight soaking means they will cook just as quickly as the finely milled ones. I make my porridge with water, which some people find really strange, but soaking the oats naturally creates a thin oat milk.

The compote can be made in advance and stored in the fridge in a tightly sealed jar for up to 10 days, as the lemon juice helps to preserve it. It's lovely with yogurt or spooned onto toast.

I hate putting hot food onto cold plates or bowls. To quickly heat a bowl, slowly pour some just-boiled water from the kettle into a room temperature bowl and leave to sit for about 30 seconds. Pour out the water, dry the bowl and add your hot food.

BLUEBERRY AND COCONUT PORRIDGE

1   Put the oats in the pot you'll cook them in, then pour over the water and allow to soak overnight.

2   The next day, bring the oats up to a simmer, stirring regularly to ensure the porridge doesn't stick to the bottom of the pot. Cook for about 6 minutes, until the porridge has thickened.

3   Meanwhile, to make the compote, put the berries, water, agave syrup or sugar and chia seeds in a small saucepan and bring to the boil. Reduce the heat and simmer for a further 2 minutes, until the sugar has dissolved and the berries are soft. Remove from the heat and stir in the lemon juice. Use the back of a fork or a potato masher to break it down to a purée. If you want it to be really smooth, transfer to a blender or use a hand-held blender and pulse until it's the consistency you want. Use immediately or allow to cool and store in a sterilised jar in the fridge. (See the note on page 30 on how to sterilise jars.)

4   When the porridge has reached a thick consistency, remove the pan from the heat and stir in the almond milk, coconut flakes or desiccated coconut and the coconut oil. Pour it into a warmed bowl, then swirl in a spoonful of compote and top with another sprinkling of coconut.

I love porridge as a warming breakfast option, but it can be a little bland. The coconut flakes in this version add a nutty taste and a bit of variety.

The key to making a quick porridge in the morning is soaking the oats overnight, which also makes it creamier. I put the oats and water right in the pot and leave it soaking on the hob before I go to bed. In the morning, I turn the hob onto the lowest heat setting while I get ready to warm up the porridge, then it just needs a quick blast of heat before I sit down to enjoy it.

Serves 1

1¾ oz (50g) jumbo oats

1 cup (250ml) filtered water

splash of almond or plant-based milk

1 tablespoon coconut flakes or
    desiccated coconut, plus extra to
    serve

1 teaspoon coconut oil

FOR THE BLUEBERRY COMPOTE:

5¼ oz (150g) fresh or frozen
    blueberries

2 tablespoons filtered water

1 tablespoon agave syrup or coconut
    sugar

1 teaspoon chia seeds

1 tablespoon fresh lemon juice

COCONUT AND ALMOND CHIA PUDDING WITH ZESTY BERRY COMPOTE

Chia pudding is the perfect on-the-go breakfast option. A small amount really fills you up, it's easy to transport in a jam jar and it's quick and easy to prepare a few jars of this for three or four days' worth of breakfasts.

Once you have the basic vanilla flavour in place, it creates the perfect canvas for adding whatever toppings you like. I love a little compote or chia jam, a swirl of almond butter and some fresh or dried berries. Other options are chopped nuts, flaked almonds, granola, flaxseed mix, coconut flakes or goji berries.

Serves 2

1 cup (250ml) almond or coconut milk (from a tin)
1 Medjool date, pitted and finely chopped, or 1 teaspoon agave syrup
4 tablespoons chia seeds
1 teaspoon desiccated coconut

FOR THE ZESTY BERRY COMPOTE:
5¼ oz (150g) fresh or frozen mixed berries
2 tablespoons freshly squeezed orange juice
1 tablespoon orange zest (optional)

1   To make the berry compote, put the berries and orange juice in a small saucepan and bring to the boil. Reduce the heat and simmer for 5 minutes, pressing the berries against the side of the pan to help break them down. Stir in the orange zest (if using) and allow to cool before transferring to a jar and storing in the fridge for up to one week.

2   To make the pudding, put the milk, chopped date or agave syrup, chia seeds and coconut in a sterilised mason jar or jam jar (see the note on page 30 on how to sterilise jars) and mix together. Let it sit for 10 minutes, then stir it again to make sure it's blended evenly. Seal the jar and put in the fridge for at least 8 hours or overnight. It will develop a jelly-like consistency. It will keep at this stage for up to three days.

3   To serve, swirl in a layer of the compote and add whatever other toppings you like (see the suggestions in the intro).

TIPS: Chia seeds are nutrient powerhouses. If you ever see them on special offer they're a worthwhile purchase, as they have a long shelf life and are so useful. If you're making this the night before, you can add frozen berries to the pudding and they will have thawed by the morning.

I generally only prep for up to four days, as I need a change after that. When I've done a week's worth of prep, inevitably some of it goes to waste due to an unforeseen change in my schedule or simply because I get bored eating the same thing.

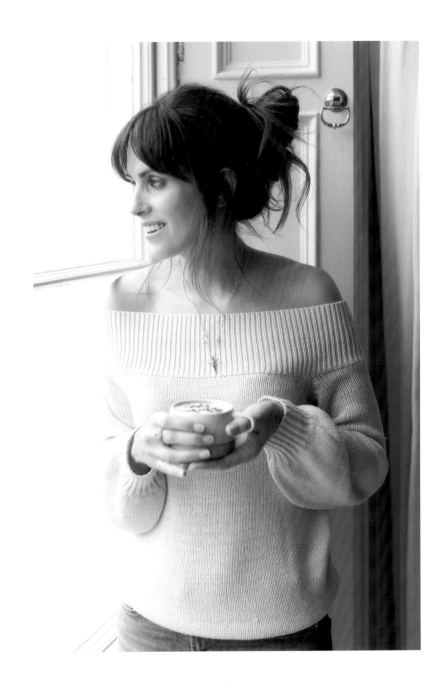

My idea of a salad used to be something that was added as a garnish to the side of a main course, and most likely left behind. Things are very different now! Salads like these are hearty, nourishing, filling and delicious. Most can be prepped in advance and are tasty enough to form a main course to suit almost any palate.

SALADS

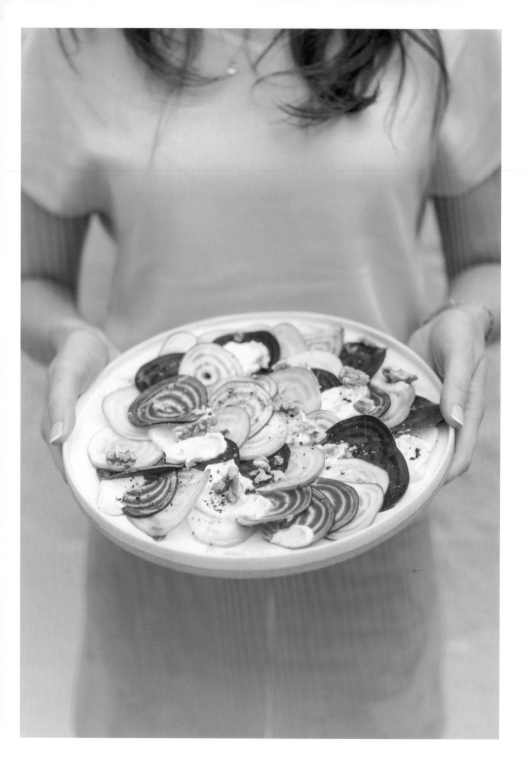

BEETROOT CARPACCIO WITH CASHEW CREAM CHEESE AND WALNUTS

1   Put the cashews in a bowl, cover with filtered water and soak for at least 8 hours or ideally overnight. Drain and rinse, then pat them dry thoroughly with a clean tea towel or kitchen paper. (See the note on page 30 on soaking nuts.)

2   Put the cashews in a high-powered blender with the remaining cream cheese ingredients. Drizzle in the water with the motor running until your desired consistency is reached. Blitz until smooth. Put in the fridge to thicken while you make your beetroot carpaccio.

3   Using a mandoline, a peeler or the thinnest setting on your food processor, cut at least four paper-thin slices of beetroot per person. Lay them out on a plate. Whisk the olive oil and lemon juice together, then massage this into each slice along with a pinch of salt. They are quite delicate, so be gentle. The salt will begin to slightly cure the beetroot and within a few minutes the texture will become much lighter.

4   Arrange the beetroot on four serving plates with a spoonful of the cream cheese and four or five walnut halves per serving. Drizzle a little agave over each dish before serving.

TIPS: You need to be extremely cautious when using a mandoline. Ensure you are in no rush whatsoever, and when you get towards the end of your veg and are getting close to the blade, set them aside for juicing and go back in with a full beetroot. Cutting your finger isn't worth it to save an inch of beetroot or carrot.

The black salt in the cashew cream cheese isn't essential, but it does make it taste very similar to regular cream cheese. You can find it in any Asian market or online.

Beetroot is one of those vegetables that everyone assumes you're happy to eat 24/7 if you're a vegan. I like beetroot in juices but find that if it's not prepared well, it can be too earthy. Here, though, it's so thinly sliced that it takes on a completely different texture. The smooth cheese, the crunch of the walnuts and the drizzle of sweet agave is a beautiful combination and makes for a stunning starter.

Serves 4

2 large beetroots, peeled
1 tablespoon olive oil
squeeze of lemon juice
a pinch of sea salt
16–20 walnut halves
drizzle of agave syrup

FOR THE CASHEW CREAM CHEESE:
3½ oz (100g) cashew nuts
approx. 4¼ fl oz (125ml) filtered water
1 tablespoon lemon juice
1 teaspoon garlic powder
½ teaspoon fine sea salt
½ teaspoon black salt

CHICKPEA, OLIVE AND SUN-DRIED TOMATO SALAD

Humble canned chickpeas are a delicious, convenient and quick lunch option.

Serves 4

1 x 14 oz (400g) tin of chickpeas, drained and rinsed

1 oz (30g) sun-dried tomatoes, chopped

¾ oz (20g) black olives, pitted and chopped

1 ripe avocado, peeled, stoned and cubed (optional)

½ red onion, finely diced (approx. 1½ oz [40g])

a handful of rocket

a handful of fresh flat-leaf parsley, chopped

sea salt and freshly ground black pepper

FOR THE DRESSING:

1 tablespoon olive oil

1 tablespoon raw apple cider vinegar

2 teaspoons tamari, soy sauce or coconut aminos

1 teaspoon wholegrain mustard (optional)

1   Put the drained and rinsed chickpeas on a clean tea towel or kitchen paper and pat them dry to absorb as much moisture as possible.

2   Put all the dressing ingredients in a large bowl and whisk to combine. Add the chickpeas, tomatoes, olives, avocado (if using), red onion, rocket and parsley (leave out the avocado and rocket if you're making this in advance). Toss to ensure everything is evenly coated in the dressing. Add salt and pepper to taste.

3   You can make this salad up to three days in advance and keep it in an airtight container in the fridge as long as you don't add the avocado or rocket until just before serving.

TIP: Only use half the amount of vinegar called for if you don't like your dressing too sharp.

TOFU TABBOULEH

1 Rinse the bulgur well, then put in a heatproof bowl and pour over the just-boiled water. Cover the bowl and set aside for about 20 minutes, until all the water has been absorbed.

2 Put the tomatoes in a sieve over a bowl with a pinch of salt and let them drain. Stir them occasionally to ensure they are draining evenly. Reserve the water to use later on.

3 Remove the tofu from the packet and pat it dry really well with kitchen paper, then chop finely.

4 Heat a little olive oil in a frying pan set over a medium heat. Add the tofu and fry for 8 minutes, stirring occasionally. Push the tofu to the side of the pan, then add the shallots and garlic and fry just until the shallots have turned transparent, then stir the tofu back in. Take the pan off the heat and stir in the miso paste, ensuring the tofu is evenly coated. Allow to cool.

5 Whisk together 2 tablespoons of the drained tomato water with the lemon juice and cumin in a large bowl. Fluff up the bulgur with a fork, then add to the bowl along with the drained tomatoes, cooled tofu mixture, spring onions and parsley. Add a little freshly ground black pepper if needed and top with the flaked almonds.

TIPS: This is a great meal prepping option, as it stays fresh for up to three days in an airtight container in the fridge. It's also an easy dish to make in advance if you've got people coming over.

If you want to scale this up, the ratio for preparing bulgur is two parts hot water to one part grain.

Tabbouleh is traditionally made with bulgur wheat, but you could just as easily make this with couscous, rice or quinoa.

Serves 4

10½ oz (300g) bulgur wheat
2½ cup (600ml) just-boiled water
3 tomatoes, cored and chopped
sea salt
1 x 14 oz (400g) block of tofu
olive oil, for frying
2 shallots, finely chopped
3 garlic cloves, crushed
1 teaspoon miso paste
juice of 2 lemons
½ teaspoon ground cumin
2 spring onions, thinly sliced
a large handful of fresh flat-leaf
 parsley, chopped
freshly ground black pepper
a handful of flaked almonds

LENTIL, TOMATO AND BULGUR SALAD

Adding lentils to this dish not only adds protein, but also gives the salad a much more interesting flavour. I've used tinned lentils here for those times when you need a quick dinner, but you could easily boil up some dried ones. It only takes 20 minutes – see the recipe on page 311.

Serves 4

1 tablespoon olive oil

1 large onion, finely diced

2 garlic cloves, crushed

½ teaspoon ground cumin

1 x 14 oz (400g) tin of chopped
    tomatoes

1 x 14 oz (400g) tin of green lentils,
    drained and rinsed

5¼ oz (150g) bulgur, rinsed

6¾ fl oz (200ml) filtered water

sea salt and freshly ground
    black pepper

1   Heat the oil in a wide-based frying pan set over a medium heat. Add the onion, garlic and cumin and fry for 8–10 minutes, until the onion has become softened and transparent. Add the tinned tomatoes and stir well to blend all the flavours, then add the lentils, rinsed bulgur and water and cover the pan with a lid.

2   Reduce the heat to a low simmer and cook for about 10 minutes. You may need to add a little more water to it. Season well with salt and pepper and serve on warmed plates.

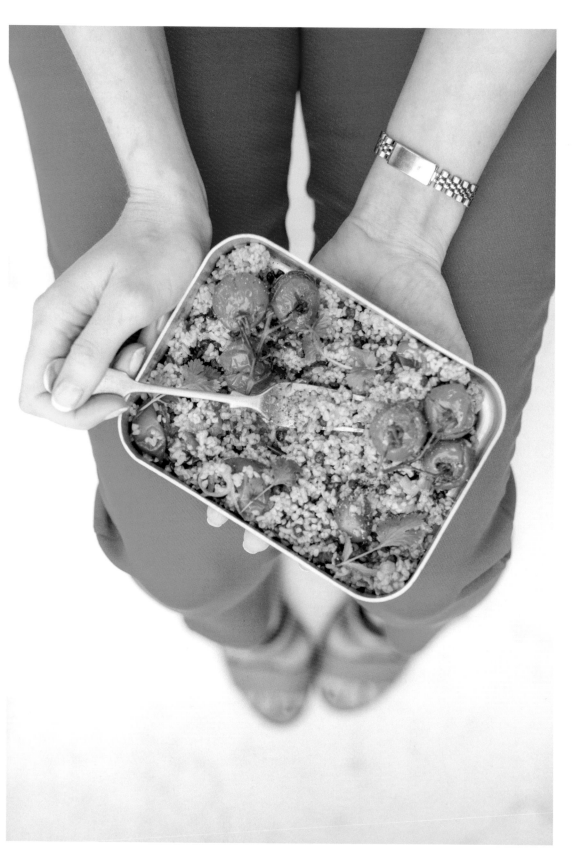

BUTTERNUT SQUASH, AVOCADO AND BLACK OLIVE SALAD WITH TAHINI DRESSING

If I'm craving something sweet and eat a dish like this, it ticks all the taste bud boxes. You need a sharp dressing to cut through the sweetness, and this tahini dressing does just that.

Serves 2

½ butternut squash (approx. 1⅓ lb [600g]), peeled and cubed
olive oil, for roasting
sea salt and freshly ground black pepper
a handful of pine nuts
2 handfuls of rocket
1 ripe avocado, peeled, stoned and sliced
20 black olives, pitted and halved
tahini dressing (page 232)

1 Preheat the oven to 350°F (170°C).
2 Put the squash on a baking tray and drizzle with a little oil. Roast in the oven for about 50 minutes, until the squash is soft and the edges are starting to turn golden. The smaller your cubes are, the quicker it will cook, so check halfway through and turn them to ensure they cook evenly. Allow to sit for about 10 minutes, then add a pinch of salt and pepper.
3 Meanwhile, put a dry frying pan over a medium heat. Add the pine nuts and cook for a few minutes, until lightly toasted. Tip out onto a plate.
4 Pile a handful of rocket on each plate and drizzle with the tahini dressing. Add the squash, avocado and olives and top with the toasted pine nuts.

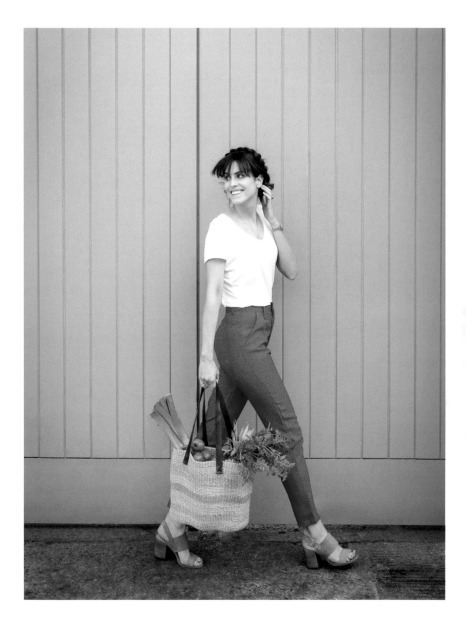

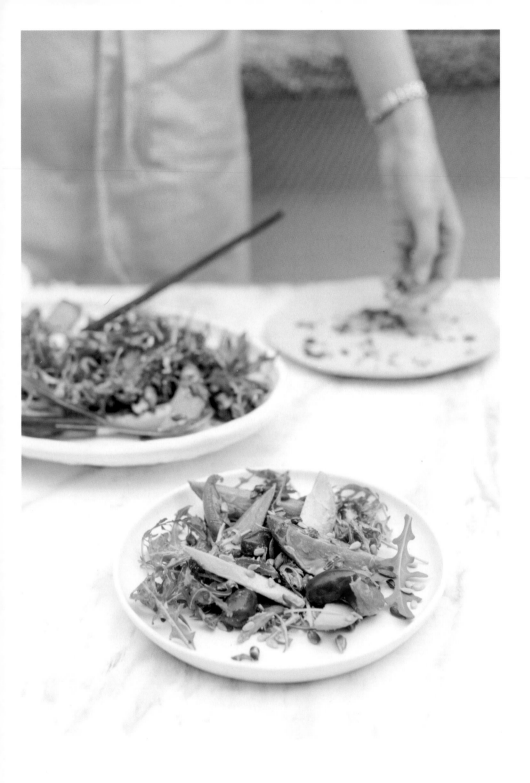

WARM SWEET POTATO, SUN-DRIED TOMATO AND ROCKET SALAD

1 Preheat the oven to 325°F (160°C).

2 Lightly dust the sweet potato cubes with a tiny bit of cornflour before placing on a baking tray and roasting in the oven for 40 minutes. Allow to cool slightly.

3 Meanwhile, make the dressing by whisking together all the ingredients except the maple syrup. If it's too sour add a tiny bit of maple syrup, but bear in mind that the sweet potatoes will balance the flavours.

4 Put the rocket on a large serving platter. Put the cooled sweet potatoes in a bowl with the sun-dried tomatoes and olives. Pour the dressing over and toss well to combine. The warmth of the potatoes will help to bring out some of the olive flavours. Arrange on top of the rocket, then scatter the sunflower and pumpkin seeds over the top.

5 Just before serving, arrange the avocado slices across the top. Serve immediately on warmed plates.

TIPS: I have this recipe for four as usually if I make this in the evening, and I like to have leftovers to eat the next day for lunch. It holds well for up to a day but not much longer, as the rocket starts to wilt. Just halve the recipe if you don't want leftovers.

I leave the skin on the sweet potatoes, but you can peel them if you like.

Squeeze a little lemon juice on the salad if you're prepping this in advance to stop the avocado turning brown.

This salad combines the perfect blend of sweet, savoury and sour flavours and also looks beautiful on a big sharing platter in the middle of a table.

Serves 4

1 lb (500g) sweet potatoes, scrubbed
   and cut into cubes
cornflour, for dusting
5¼ oz (150g) rocket
1¾ oz (50g) sun-dried tomatoes,
   sliced
1¾ oz (50g) black olives, pitted and
   halved
1¾ oz (50g) sunflower seeds
1¾ oz (50g) pumpkin seeds
1 ripe avocado, peeled, stoned
   and sliced

FOR THE DRESSING:
juice of 1 lemon
1 tablespoon olive oil
1 tablespoon tahini
1 teaspoon tamari, soy sauce
   or coconut aminos
sea salt and freshly ground
   black pepper
drizzle of maple syrup (optional)

I typically eat light during the day as I'm
on the go, so I don't want to spend too long
preparing anything. These are all quick and
easy to assemble lunch options that are not only
nourishing they're creative and delicious too.

LUNCHES

ROASTED TOMATO, SQUASH AND CHILLI SOUP

I wish I had a warming, hearty soup on the stove all the time. This has so much flavour but is incredibly simple to make. A bit of chopping is involved initially, but once it's in the oven it needs very little attention.

Serves 5

1 lb (500g) ripe tomatoes, chopped

10½ oz (300g) butternut squash, peeled and chopped

2 onions, chopped

1 garlic clove, chopped

1 fresh red chilli, deseeded and roughly chopped

a large sprig of fresh thyme

olive oil, for roasting

sea salt and freshly ground black pepper

2 cup (500ml) vegetable stock (page 303)

½ x approx. 1¾ cup (400ml) tin of coconut milk

fresh chopped cilantro, to garnish

1 Preheat the oven to 350°F (180°C).

2 Put all the vegetables and the sprig of thyme in a roasting tin. Drizzle with a little olive oil and season with salt and pepper, then roast in the oven for about 30 minutes, until tender. Remove the thyme stalk.

3 Transfer the vegetables to a blender or a large pot if using a hand-held blender. Add the vegetable stock and blend to your desired consistency. Stir in the coconut milk and serve in warmed bowls with freshly chopped cilantro on top.

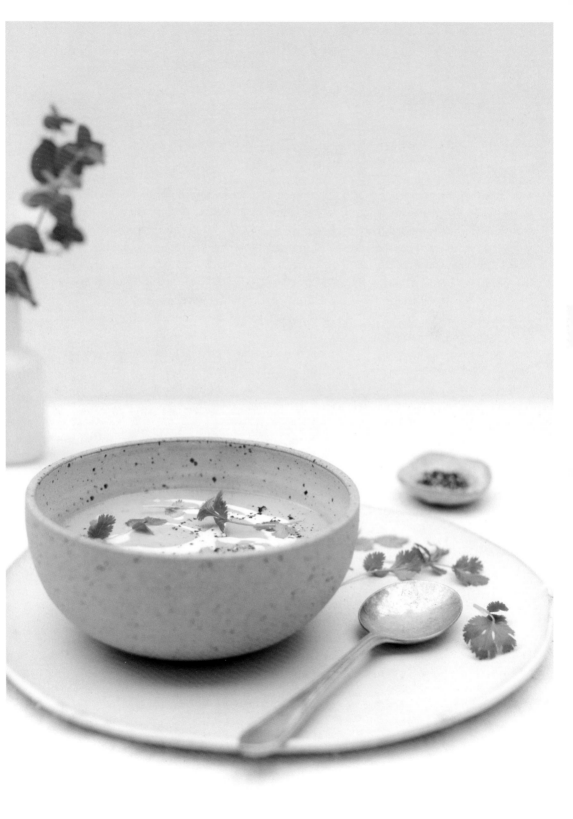

MISO SOUP WITH TOFU AND VEGETABLES

In Asian restaurants miso soup is often quite thin, with a scattering of spring onions, some seaweed and tofu. I like to load it up with more vegetables to make it more of a meal in itself rather than an addition to one. This blend of mushrooms, carrots and courgettes makes for quite a hearty option that tides you over between meals or is more than sufficient on those days when you want something light and nourishing. In fact, a good miso soup replicates the soothing qualities of chicken soup on a vegan diet.

Serves 4

FOR THE DASHI (STOCK):

4¼ cup (1 litre) filtered water

1 x 2" (5cm) strip of kombu seaweed

1 dried shiitake mushroom

FOR THE SOUP:

olive oil, for cooking

7 oz (200g) button mushrooms, sliced

1 carrot, peeled and thinly sliced

1 courgette, peeled and finely sliced

1 tablespoon dried wakame seaweed

½ x 14 oz (400g) block of tofu, cubed

3 spring onions, finely chopped

2 heaped tablespoons miso paste

1 To make the dashi, put the filtered water, kombu seaweed and dried shiitake mushroom in a large saucepan and bring to the boil, then reduce the heat and simmer for 10 minutes. Remove the kombu and discard.

2 Heat a little olive oil in a separate pan set over a medium heat. Add the button mushrooms, carrot and courgette and lightly sauté for about 10 minutes, until they are beginning to soften.

3 Transfer the sautéed vegetables to the saucepan with the dashi and add the dried wakame seaweed too. Cook over a medium heat for about 5 minutes, although the longer you simmer the wakame, the less of a salty, fishy flavour it will have. Wakame expands as it cooks, so don't overload the pan with it or add any more until you see how big it has gotten.

4 Reduce the heat to very low, then add the tofu, spring onions and miso paste, stirring until the miso has dissolved. Don't boil the soup after adding the miso, as it's a live culture and boiling it will ruin its beneficial properties and change the flavour of the soup. Serve warm, never piping hot.

TIP: You can find miso and tofu in most supermarkets. Kombu and wakame are available in Asian markets, artisan and health food stores. Each bag of seaweed will be enough for several batches and it has a long shelf life, so they're handy additions to have in your press.

TOFU CLUB SANDWICH

1 First you need to press the tofu. To do this, put the tofu on a chopping board with at least four layers of kitchen paper above and below it, then wrap it up in a clean tea towel. Put a plate on top of the towel, then add a weight to the plate – a tin of beans works well. The weight will press some of the excess moisture out of the tofu, giving it a firmer texture and also enabling it to absorb more of the flavours you marinate it in. Leave it for at least 30 minutes, then unwrap the tofu and pat it dry. The amount of moisture released will surprise you!

2 Cut the block of tofu lengthways into thin slices so that they will fit into your sandwich easily. I usually aim to cut a 14 oz (400g) block into eight slices.

3 Whisk together the garlic, soy sauce and vinegar in an airtight container, then add the tofu slices and cover with the lid. Leave to marinate for as long as possible – overnight is ideal.

4 When you're ready to make the sandwiches, slice the tomato, scatter over a pinch of salt and leave it to drain in a sieve set over a bowl. This prevents your sandwich going soggy, so don't be tempted to skip this useful step.

5 Heat a little olive oil in a chargrill pan set over a high heat. Put the tofu in the hot pan and cook for 6–8 minutes, until nice char marks form. Carefully turn the tofu over and cook the other side for a further 5 minutes, again until char marks form.

6 Meanwhile, toast your bread and slice your avocado. Drizzle a little fresh lemon juice on it straight away to stop it turning brown.

(continued)

The secret to this is marinating the tofu, ideally overnight. Once that and your mayonnaise are right, the rest will fall into place.

Serves 2

1 x 14 oz (400g) block of tofu

1 garlic clove, crushed, or ½ teaspoon garlic powder

1 tablespoon soy sauce

1½ teaspoons raw apple cider vinegar

1 ripe tomato

sea salt and freshly ground black pepper

olive oil, for cooking

4 slices of sourdough bread

1 ripe avocado, peeled, stoned and sliced

squeeze of lemon juice

2 tablespoons vegan aioli or garlic mayonnaise (page 237)

a handful of rocket or baby spinach

7   Spread two slices of the toast with the vegan aioli or garlic mayonnaise. Add some rocket or spinach, a few avocado slices and then the tomato slices. Remove your tofu from the pan and allow it to rest for a minute before putting it on top of the tomato. Sprinkle with a little salt and pepper.

8   Add the remaining slices of toast on top and firmly press them down. Use a cocktail stick to hold the sandwich together and serve immediately.

TIPS: I love good sourdough for this sandwich, as once toasted it's very firm and will hold the contents nicely.

If you have one, use an egg slicer to cut the avocado.

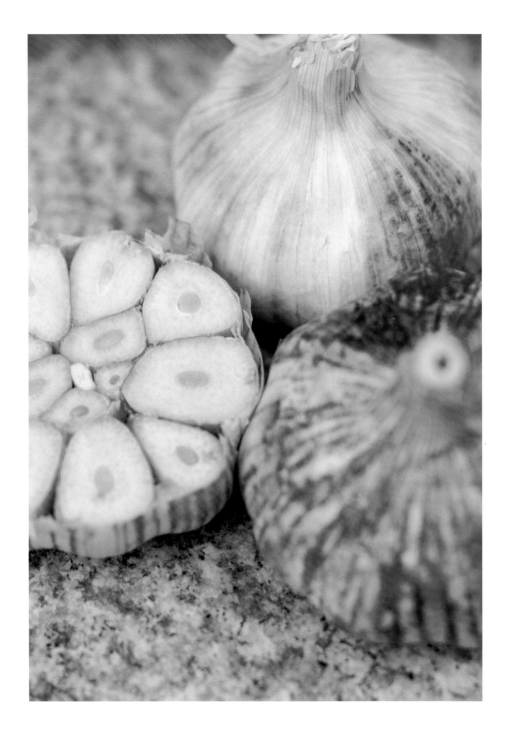

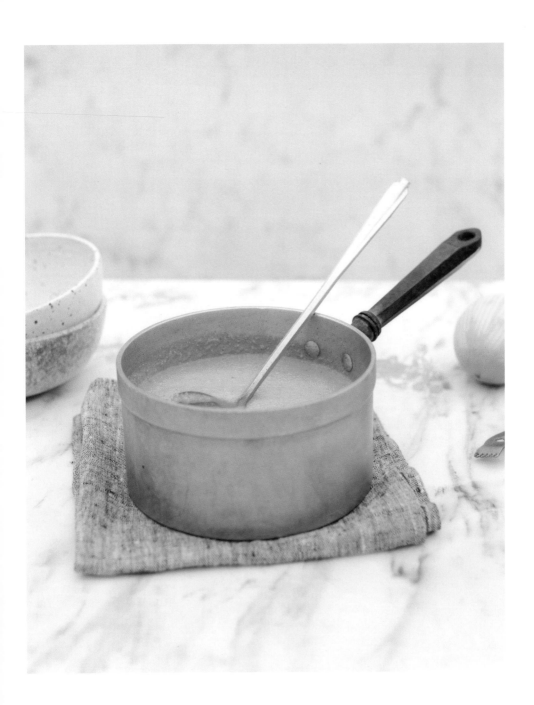

CAULIFLOWER AND SQUASH BISQUE

1 Put the cashews in a bowl, cover with filtered water and soak for at least 8 hours or ideally overnight. Drain and rinse, then pat them dry thoroughly with a clean tea towel or kitchen paper. (See the note on page 30 on soaking nuts.)

2 Preheat the oven to 285°F (140°C).

3 Put the squash on a baking tray, cut side down. Add the cauliflower, onion and garlic and drizzle with olive oil. Roast in the oven for about 1 hour, until tender. Allow the squash to cool before scooping out the flesh into a blender or a pot if you'll be using a hand-held blender. Discard the skin.

4 Squeeze the garlic out of its skins into the blender or pot. Add the roasted cauliflower and onion along with the soaked cashews, stock, turmeric and miso. Blend to a smooth, thick consistency and simmer until you're ready to serve.

5 To serve, ladle into warmed bowls, then sprinkle on the lemon zest and add a drizzle of truffle or olive oil.

This is a thick and incredibly comforting soup that I really love. Roasting the vegetables and the garlic beforehand brings a richness to it that you can really taste and the miso balances out the sweetness of the squash perfectly.

Serves 4

1½ oz (40g) cashew nuts

½ butternut squash (approx. 14 oz [400g]), seeds scraped out

1 head of cauliflower, broken into florets

1 large white onion, cut into quarters

3 garlic cloves, unpeeled

olive oil, for drizzling

3⅓ cup (800ml) vegetable stock (page 303)

1 teaspoon ground turmeric

1 teaspoon white miso paste

1 teaspoon lemon zest

a drizzle of truffle oil, to serve

BROCCOLI, PEA AND LEEK SOUP WITH ROASTED GARLIC CIABATTA

The cashews add a creaminess that elevates vegan soups to a luxurious territory that you might not have thought possible.

Serves 4

1¾ oz (50g) cashews

14 oz (400g) broccoli or broccolini

1 tablespoon olive oil

1 onion, chopped

2 garlic cloves, chopped

2 leeks, chopped

1 courgette, thinly sliced

7 oz (200g) fresh or frozen peas

4¼ cup (1 litre) vegetable stock (page 303)

FOR THE ROASTED GARLIC CIABATTA:

1 head of garlic

2 teaspoons olive oil

1 loaf of ciabatta bread, sliced and toasted

1   Put the cashews in a bowl, cover with filtered water and soak for at least 8 hours or ideally overnight. Drain and rinse, then pat them dry thoroughly with a clean tea towel or kitchen paper. (See the note on page 30 on soaking nuts.)

2   Preheat the oven to 350°F (170°C).

3   Remove the papery outer layer of skin from the head of garlic, leaving the head itself intact with all the cloves still connected. Trim about ¼" (5mm) off the top of the head of garlic to expose the tops of the cloves. Put the garlic on a large piece of foil, then drizzle the oil over the top and tightly seal up the foil. Roast the garlic in the oven for 40–50 minutes.

4   Meanwhile, break up the broccoli into florets. If you're using broccolini, cut it into a few pieces, stems and all.

5   Heat the oil in a saucepan set over a high heat. Add the broccoli, onion and garlic and sauté for 4–5 minutes, until softened.

6   Add the leeks, courgette, peas and 2 tablespoons of the stock. Reduce the heat to medium and put on the lid. Cook for about 15 minutes, until the vegetables have started to soften.

7   Put the soaked cashews in a high-powered blender with a little stock and blitz until smooth. Add the vegetables and pulse to combine, then pour in the rest of the stock. Purée the soup to your preference – I don't like to fully blend it, as I like a little bit of texture. Keep it warm until ready to serve.

8   Take the garlic out of the oven and carefully open the foil parcel, watching out for the hot steam that might escape. Squeeze the roasted garlic into a little bowl to be spread on the toasted ciabatta and dunked into the soup.

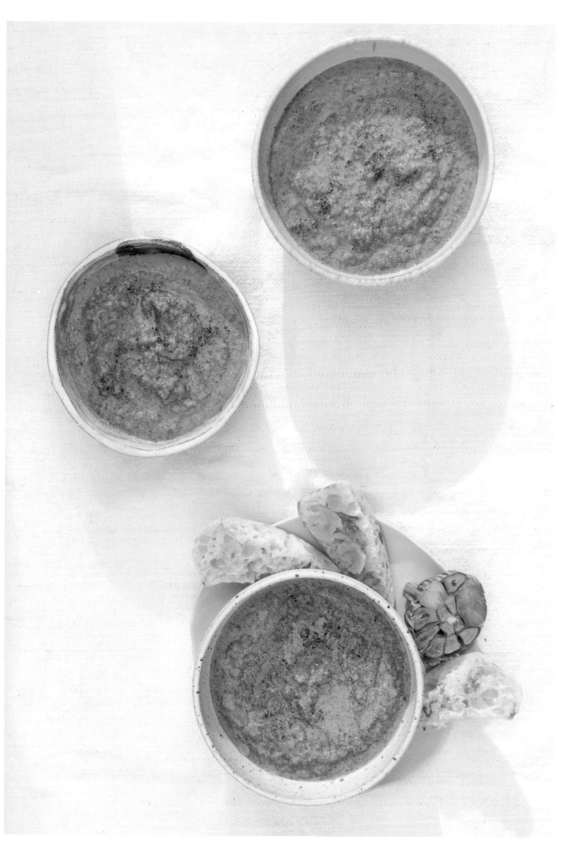

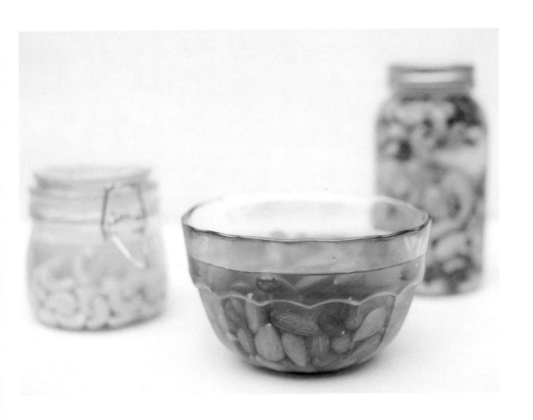

BAKED SWEET POTATOES WITH CASHEW CHEESE AND OLIVES

1   Preheat the oven to 300°F (150°C).

2   Scrub your potatoes clean and prick each one a few times with a fork so they don't explode while cooking. Put on a baking tray and roast in the oven for about an hour, until cooked through.

3   Cut a slit on top of each sweet potato, drizzle with a little olive oil and fluff up the inside with a fork. Put on warmed plates, then top with the cashew cheese and season with salt and cayenne pepper to taste. Squeeze the lemon juice over the potatoes, scatter over the olives and garnish with sprouts and seeds.

TIP: Serve the baked potatoes with a green salad for a light bite or with tofu steaks, roasted vegetables or one-pot ratatouille (page 123) for a more filling dinner.

You can use any kind of potatoes here, but the cashew cheese goes exceptionally well with sweet potatoes.
Serves 1

1 large or 2 small sweet potatoes
    per person
olive oil, for drizzling
cashew cheese (page 305), to serve
a pinch of sea salt
a pinch of cayenne pepper
1 lemon, cut into wedges
1 oz (30g) Kalamata olives, pitted
    and sliced
sprouts and seeds, to garnish

ROASTED VEGETABLE BUDDHA BOWL

This is essentially a combination of lots of side dishes that all come together to form a quick dinner or lunch. Use whatever you have to hand, and as long as you adhere to the basic combination of carbs, proteins, greens and healthy fats, usually in the form of a dressing and nuts, this will be a balanced meal for any time of day. I typically combine some roasted sweet potatoes, kale with roasted chickpeas and tahini dressing (page 157), brown rice with miso (page 150) and marinated tofu with whatever leaves or vegetables I might have.

Makes 4

2 red peppers, sliced

2 courgettes, cut into half-moons

2 sweet potatoes, cut into cubes

2 red onions, finely chopped

olive oil

1 x 14 oz (400g) tin of chickpeas, drained, rinsed and dried

1 teaspoon ground cumin

1 teaspoon dried oregano

8½ oz (240g) quinoa

2 ripe avocados, peeled, stoned and sliced

4 tablespoons hummus

4 tablespoons miso dressing (page 233)

a handful of chopped almonds

1 Preheat the oven to 350°F (180°C).

2 Put all the vegetables in a roasting tin, drizzle with 1 tablespoon of olive oil and toss to coat. Roast in the oven for 40 minutes, until tender.

3 Toss the chickpeas in 1½ teaspoons of olive oil along with the cumin and oregano. Tip out onto a baking tray and put in the oven along with the vegetables to roast for 40 minutes too.

4 Meanwhile, cook the quinoa as per the packet instructions or follow my instructions on how to cook quinoa on page 312. Put 2–3 tablespoons of cooked quinoa in the bottom of each warmed serving bowl as your base layer.

5 Once cooked, allow the vegetables and chickpeas to cool for 5 minutes before adding to the serving bowls on top of the quinoa. Add the avocado slices, then top each bowl with a tablespoon of hummus and a drizzle of miso dressing, then scatter with chopped almonds.

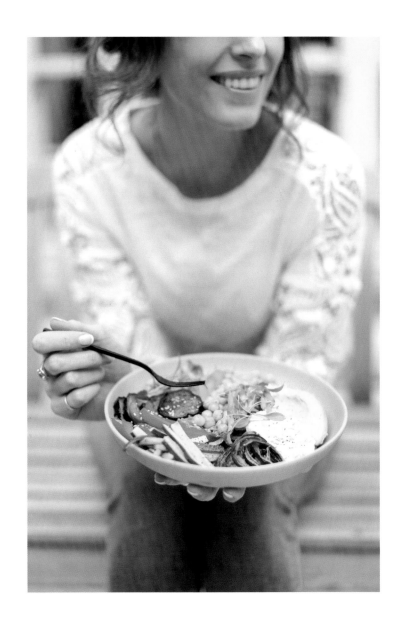

GRILLED COURGETTE, AVOCADO AND PESTO TOASTIE

I guarantee that you will never have a nicer sandwich than this!

Makes 1

½ courgette

olive oil, for frying

2 slices of sourdough or rye bread, toasted

1 tablespoon vegan pesto (page 239)

½ ripe avocado, peeled, stoned and sliced

3 cherry tomatoes, sliced (optional)

a small handful of rocket or baby spinach

1 Using a mandoline or vegetable peeler, peel the courgette into thin ribbons.

2 Heat some olive oil in a chargrill pan set over a high heat. Add the courgette ribbons to the hot pan and sear for about 1 minute on each side, until nice char marks form.

3 Spread one slice of toast with the pesto, then add the avocado slices, grilled courgette ribbons, cherry tomatoes (if using) and rocket or spinach. Top with the second slice of toast, cut in half on the diagonal and eat straight away, while still warm.

TIP: Sourdough is great for sandwiches as it stays firm once toasted, so you can really load it up, but rye bread works well too.

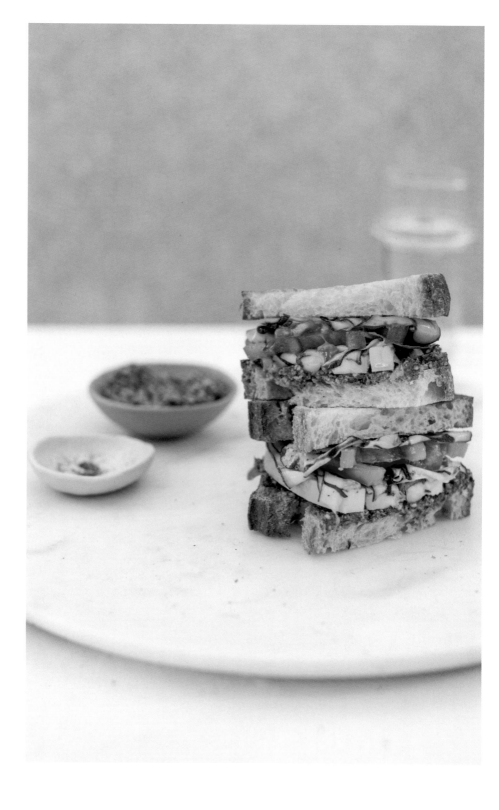

My evening meal is usually my largest and the one I can spend a bit more time preparing. At the end of the day, I love turning on a podcast and immersing myself in a bit of cooking. I tend to make larger portions and often make enough for two nights or for leftovers for lunch the next day – so feel free to double up!

MAINS

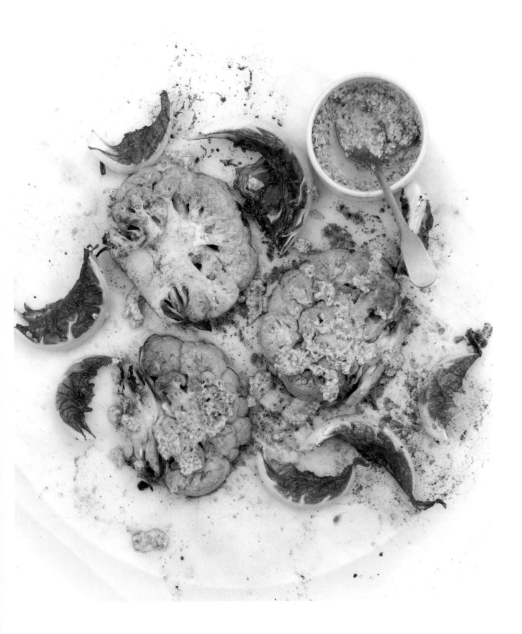

ROASTED CAULIFLOWER STEAKS WITH GARLIC SAUCE

1   Preheat the oven to 350°F (180°C). Line two large baking trays with non-stick baking paper or brush with a little olive oil.

2   Wash the cauliflower and remove the outer leaves. Slice each cauliflower into four 'steaks' about 1" (2.5cm) thick. Put the steaks on the prepared baking trays.

3   Mix the spices with a drizzle of olive oil in a small bowl. Using a pastry brush or a spoon, coat both sides of the steaks as evenly as possible with the spices.

4   Roast in the oven for 30 minutes, turning the cauliflower midway through to make sure it cooks evenly and doesn't burn. I like it to be as crisp as possible, so I put it under the grill for a quick 1-minute blast at the end.

5   While the cauliflower is roasting, make the sauce by blending all the ingredients with half of the water to form a thick paste. Depending on whether you want a thick dip or a runny sauce to drizzle over the steaks, add more water to thin the sauce to your desired consistency.

6   When your cauliflower is crisp, remove it from the oven, put on warmed plates and season with salt and pepper. Pour the sauce over or serve it on the side. This can be served hot or cold and holds well in the fridge for up to three days.

TIP: If you are prepping this in advance, you can let the steaks marinate in the fridge with the spice seasoning to enhance the flavours.

Roasted cauliflower is one of those surprising discoveries that's a million miles away from the bland steamed cauliflower we were served in boarding school. In order for the cauliflower steaks to get nice and crisp they need to be as dry as possible, so after you wash them, put them on a piece of kitchen paper or a clean tea towel and pat them dry to absorb as much moisture as possible.

Serves 4

2 heads of cauliflower
olive oil, for greasing and roasting
1 teaspoon ground cumin
1 teaspoon ground turmeric
½ teaspoon paprika
½ teaspoon garlic powder
sea salt and freshly ground
    black pepper

FOR THE GARLIC SAUCE:
3½ oz (100g) sesame seeds
1 shallot, finely chopped
1 garlic clove, minced
1 cup (250ml) filtered water
1 tablespoon nutritional yeast
1 tablespoon raw apple cider vinegar
1 tablespoon olive oil
a pinch of sea salt

SPIRALIZED COURGETTI WITH ROASTED TOMATOES

For a while courgetti were a big thing on Instagram and I bought into it, but initially I hated the taste. People suggested cooking them or serving them like pasta, but I didn't like those methods either. After a lot of research, I now make them this way at all my demonstrations as a gentle introduction to eating raw food and I'm always amazed by the response. So many people say that this is their favourite dish of all the ones they have tasted.

Because this is such a simple dish, the quality of the ingredients will really show. Use a good-quality extra virgin olive oil and Maldon flaky sea salt. If you don't have a spiralizer, many supermarkets now sell pre-packed spiralized veg.

Serves 1 as a main or 2 as a side

6 ripe cherry tomatoes

1 tablespoon olive oil, plus extra for
  roasting

sea salt and freshly ground black
  pepper

1 tablespoon pine nuts

1 courgette

1 garlic clove, minced

a few fresh basil leaves, to serve

1   Preheat the oven to 285°F (140°C). Line a baking tray with non-stick baking paper.
2   Put the cherry tomatoes on the lined tray. If they are large, slice them in half to speed up the cooking time. Drizzle with a little olive oil and season with a pinch of salt and pepper. Roast in the oven for about 45 minutes, until they are soft and the skins have burst.
3   Meanwhile, put a dry frying pan over a medium heat. Add the pine nuts and cook for a few minutes, until lightly toasted. Transfer to a plate and set aside.
4   Spiralize the courgette, then put it in a mixing bowl with the garlic and a pinch of salt to draw out some of the moisture from the 'noodles'. You will notice their texture change within a minute or two as they soften.
5   Drizzle over the olive oil and season with a pinch of pepper, then toss to coat the noodles in the oil. Stir in the tomatoes and toasted pine nuts. Transfer to a warmed shallow bowl and garnish with a few fresh basil leaves.

TIP: If you're preparing this in advance, don't add any salt or the oil until just before serving. It can be quickly tossed together and will taste fresher.

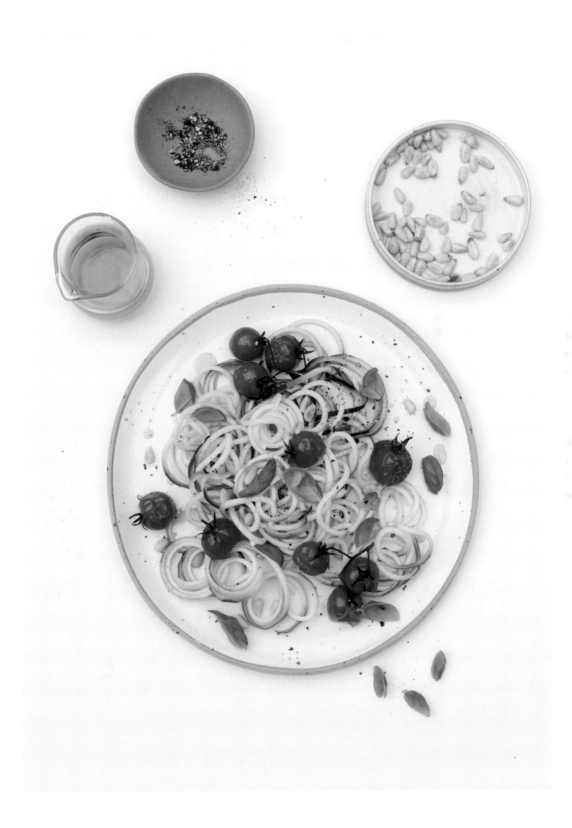

SWEET POTATO AND BUTTER BEAN STEW

Stews and casseroles are perfect warming comfort food. They also work really well in a slow cooker, which I'm convinced are going to have a revival soon. There's a bit of chopping involved, but there's no need to chase perfection. Some chunky vegetables make this more hearty.

Serves 4

2 tablespoons olive oil

1¾ lb (800g) sweet potatoes, peeled and chopped into small cubes

2 onions, finely chopped

4 garlic cloves, crushed

1 teaspoon ground cumin

1 teaspoon ground coriander

1 teaspoon smoked paprika

2 x 14 oz (400g) tins of chopped tomatoes

2 cup (500ml) vegetable stock (page 303)

2 x 14 oz (400g) tins of butter beans, drained and rinsed

sea salt and freshly ground black pepper

1 large bunch of fresh cilantro, chopped

brown rice, to serve

coconut yogurt (page 52 or 54), to serve

1   Heat the oil in a casserole set over a medium heat. Add the chopped sweet potatoes, onion, garlic and spices. Cook, stirring occasionally, for about 8 minutes, until all the flavours have combined and the potatoes have a slight golden edge.

2   Add the tinned tomatoes and stock. Bring to the boil, then reduce the heat and simmer with the lid half off for about 25 minutes, until the sweet potatoes are tender.

3   Add the butter beans and cook for another 5 minutes to warm them through. Season with salt and pepper and sprinkle over the chopped fresh cilantro leaves.

4   Serve in warmed shallow bowls with steaming bowls of brown rice and a little coconut yogurt on the side.

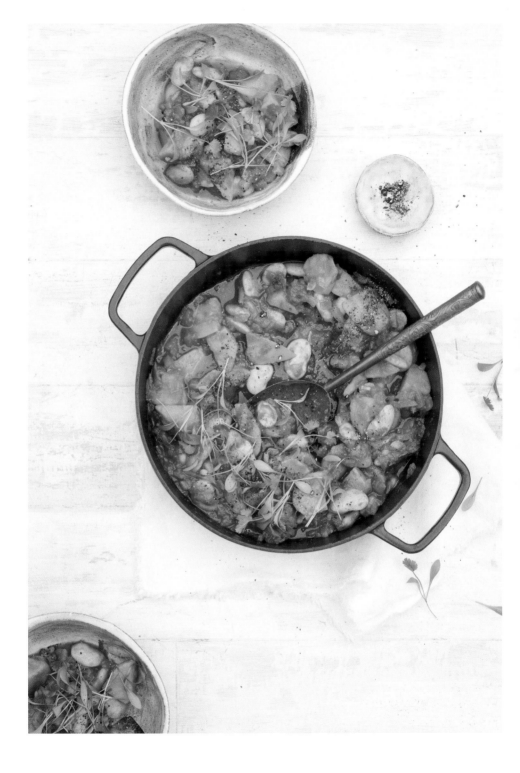

CURRIED LENTIL STEW

I'm always looking for easy, filling main courses, and since lentils contain more protein than beef, gram for gram, it's worth finding ways to integrate them into your diet. I made this at my very first demonstration, and when I came off the stage my family and in-laws, who had kindly come to support me and make sure there were actually people in the audience, all dug in to this.

Serves 4

1 vegan stock cube

olive oil, for frying

1 large carrot, chopped

1 courgette, chopped

2 garlic cloves, minced

1 teaspoon curry powder

approx. 8¾ oz (250g) dried black
   lentils, soaked and rinsed, or 2 x
   14 oz (400g) tins of black lentils,
   drained and rinsed

1 x approx. 1¾ cup (400ml) tin of
   coconut milk

4 kaffir lime leaves

1 tablespoon miso paste

sea salt and freshly ground black
   pepper

chopped fresh cilantro, to garnish

1   Dissolve the stock cube in approx. 1¼ cup (300ml) of just-boiled water. If you're using tinned lentils, use only 150ml of water.

2   Heat a little olive oil in a large saucepan set over a medium heat. Add the carrot, courgette and garlic and fry for a minute to release the flavours and soften the veg, then add the curry powder. Add the lentils and stir to mix the flavours evenly.

3   Add the stock, put on the lid and simmer for 5 minutes. Add the coconut milk and lime leaves and leave to simmer for another 5 minutes. Reduce the heat and stir in the miso paste, then take out the lime leaves. Allow to simmer on a low temperature for a further 10 minutes before seasoning to taste with salt and pepper.

4   Just before serving in warmed shallow bowls, top with some fresh chopped cilantro. This is lovely with a bitter rocket salad and some roasted cauliflower on the side.

TIPS: Most health food or gourmet food stores sell black lentils, but you could easily substitute green or brown here, which are widely available.

   You can bulk cook this and it also tastes nice cold if you want to have it as an on-the-go lunch.

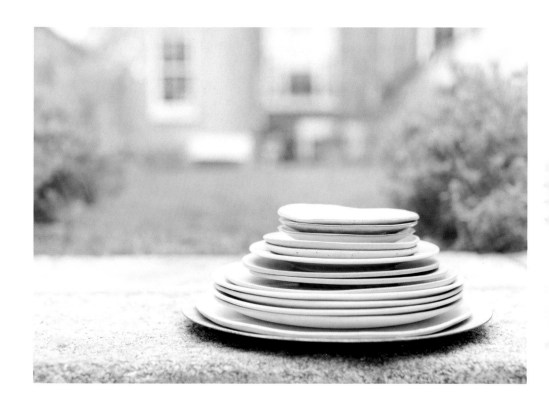

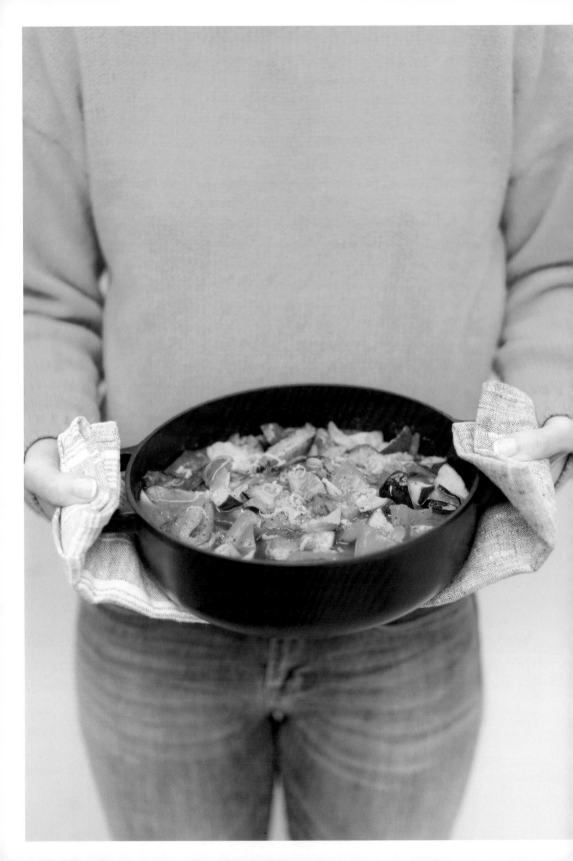

ONE-POT RATATOUILLE

1   If you have time, chop the aubergines, put them in a colander set over a bowl and sprinkle with some fine sea salt or Himalayan pink salt while you prep the rest of the ingredients. After about 20 minutes, water will have drained off them and they will have beads of water on them. Pat the aubergines with kitchen paper to dry them and to remove the salt.

2   Heat some olive oil in a casserole set over a high heat. Add the aubergines, courgettes and peppers and cook for about 8 minutes, until softened. Set them aside in a bowl.

3   Pour a little more olive oil into the casserole if needed. Add the fresh tomatoes, onions and garlic and cook for 15 minutes. Return the aubergines, courgettes and peppers to the casserole and stir to combine.

4   Stir in the tinned chopped tomatoes, herbs, wine or vinegar and the mustard. Put the lid on the casserole and let it simmer for 30 minutes. Allow to cool down for a few minutes before serving in warmed bowls with some torn fresh basil leaves and lemon zest scattered on top. Serve with thick slices of crusty bread to mop up all the sauce.

TIP: Instead of simmering this on the hob, you could finish it in the oven at 300°F (150°C) for the same amount of time.

One of the things I love about ratatouille is that it's a very mainstream vegan main course. When I went to Paris a few years back, this was widely available, satisfying and incredibly comforting.

Serves 4

2 aubergines (approx. 1¾ lb [800g])
fine sea salt or Himalayan pink salt
olive oil
2 courgettes (approx. 1 lb [500g]), cut
   into half-moons
2 red peppers (approx. 12½ oz
   [350g]), sliced into strips
6 ripe tomatoes, quartered
2 red onions, thinly sliced
4 garlic cloves, crushed
1 x 14 oz (400g) tin of chopped
   tomatoes
a few sprigs of fresh thyme
a few sprigs of fresh rosemary
3⅓ fl oz (100ml) red wine or 1
   tablespoon balsamic vinegar
½ teaspoon Dijon mustard
½ oz (15g) fresh basil, torn, to garnish
zest of ½ lemon, to garnish
crusty bread, to serve

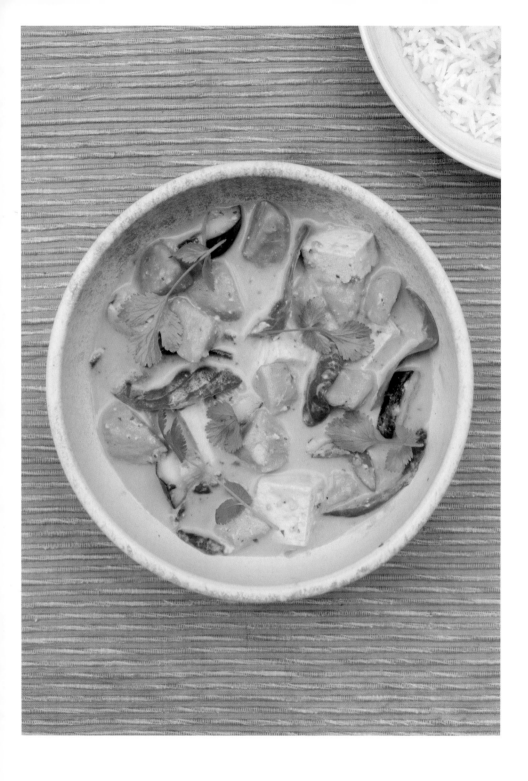

SWEET POTATO CURRY

1 Make the curry paste by blending all the ingredients together in a food processor.

2 Cook the rice as per the packet instructions. Marinate the tofu slices in the tamari while you get started on the rest of the curry. Dissolve the stock cube in 3⅓ fl oz (100ml) of just-boiled water.

3 Melt some coconut or groundnut oil in a wok or large wide-brimmed saucepan set over a medium heat. Add the sweet potato first to it to give it a head start. After about 8 minutes, when it's starting to turn golden, add the tofu as well as the tamari it was marinating in, the courgette and the red onion and lightly fry for about 5 minutes. Add 2 tablespoons of the curry paste and stir to blend evenly, then add the stock. Simmer for a further 5 minutes – the stock will have evaporated and the vegetables will have softened.

4 Add the coconut milk and simmer for 10 minutes. Just before serving, stir in the spinach and allow it to wilt. Serve in warmed shallow bowls over the jasmine rice.

TIP: This recipe makes more curry paste than you'll need, but the leftovers will keep in the fridge in a tightly sealed jam jar for up to six months or in the freezer for up to a year. Having the paste made in advance means that as long as you choose vegetables that will cook quickly or chop them finely, this can be a speedy meal.

A good curry recipe is an essential part of any plant-based kitchen. It's also a fail-safe take-away option, as most of the flavour is in the sauce and Asian restaurants tend to have plenty of tofu to offer as a meat substitute.

Serves 4

½ x 14 oz (400g) block of firm tofu, sliced

1 tablespoon tamari, soy sauce or coconut aminos

½ vegan stock cube

coconut or groundnut oil, for frying

7 oz (200g) sweet potato, peeled and cut into cubes

1 courgette, cut into half-moons

1 red onion, finely chopped

2 tablespoons curry paste

1 x approx. 1¾ cup (400ml) tin of coconut milk

a handful of baby spinach

jasmine rice, to serve

FOR THE CURRY PASTE:

a handful of fresh cilantro leaves, chopped

3 shallots, chopped

2 garlic cloves, chopped

2 sticks of lemongrass, chopped

1 fresh red chilli, deseeded and chopped

1 x 1" (2.5cm) piece of fresh ginger, peeled and chopped

3 kaffir lime leaves

1 teaspoon ground cumin

½ teaspoon ground black pepper

a pinch of sea salt

MARINATED TOFU

There are two types of tofu: silken and firm. Silken tofu is perfect for blending, but if you want it to keep its shape for frying, you need the firm variety. I always marinate a full block to have it ready in the fridge for a quick addition to a stir-fry.

Serves 4

1 x 14 oz (400g) block of firm tofu

2 tablespoons miso paste

2 tablespoons tamari, soy sauce or coconut aminos

2 tablespoons sesame oil

coconut or groundnut oil, for frying

brown rice with miso (page 150), to serve

chargrilled green beans with caramelised onions and garlic (page 151), to serve

1   First you need to press the tofu. To do this, put the tofu on a chopping board with at least four layers of kitchen paper above and below it, then wrap it up in a clean tea towel. Put a plate on top of the towel, then add a weight to the plate – a tin of beans works well. The weight will press some of the excess moisture out of the tofu, giving it a firmer texture and also enabling it to absorb more of the flavours you marinate it in. Leave it for at least 30 minutes, then unwrap the tofu and pat it dry. The amount of moisture released will surprise you!

2   Slice the tofu into whatever shape you would like to serve it in. Cutting it diagonally into triangles and then cutting it in half again is easy to manage when frying.

3   Whisk together the miso, tamari and the sesame oil in an airtight container, then add the tofu. Turn it on all sides to ensure it's well coated, cover with the lid and put in the fridge to marinate for at least 1 hour.

4   Heat a little coconut or groundnut oil in a non-stick frying pan set over a medium-high heat. Add the drained tofu and fry for about 10 minutes on each side, until golden and starting to crisp in places.

5   Serve it however you like, but I love it with miso brown rice and garlicky green beans.

MUSHROOM AND TOFU STIR-FRY WITH MISO DRESSING

There are a few secrets for stir-frying that will elevate it from something soggy and unappealing to something crisp, quick, delicious and full of flavour.

First, you need a large wok so that you can quickly move the contents of the pan around (or, for the slightly more adventurous, flip and toss the ingredients!).

Second, you need to use vegetable or groundnut oil, which has a high smoke point and can take the high heat required to crisp things up.

Have all your ingredients chopped and ready to go so that you can focus on the cooking, which happens quickly.

Last, keep the portions in the wok small to allow every ingredient to get the heat it needs. Overloading the wok and not getting the oil hot enough lead to a soggy, limp stir-fry, so it's worth being a little patient with it.

Serves 2

(continued)

1 x 14 oz (400g) block of tofu, cut into cubes

groundnut oil, for frying

1 large carrot, chopped

1 large courgette, halved lengthways and sliced into half-moons

approx. 8¾ oz (250g) pak choi, cut into 1" (2.5cm) pieces

3½ oz (100g) button or oyster mushrooms, halved

2 shallots, finely chopped

2 garlic cloves, crushed

1 x 1" (2.5cm) piece of fresh ginger, peeled and grated

a handful of baby spinach

1 batch of miso dressing (page 233)

brown rice with miso (page 150), to serve

1 Prep all your vegetables before you start to cook.

2 Remove the tofu from the packaging and put it on a piece of kitchen paper to drain a little. This stir-fry will taste even better if you marinate the tofu for an hour beforehand, using the recipe on page 126, but it's not essential.

3 Add a little groundnut oil to a large wok set over a high heat and leave it for at least a minute to really heat up. Add the tofu, carrot and courgette first and keep them moving around the wok for 1 minute. Add the pak choi, mushrooms, shallots, garlic and ginger and cook for 2 minutes, still moving everything around the wok constantly, then add the spinach, which will quickly wilt.

4 Reduce the heat and pour over the miso dressing. Add the brown rice to the wok and stir to combine all the ingredients. Cook for 1 further minute before serving in warmed shallow bowls.

TIP: You don't need to be too particular with the vegetables you use in this. The miso dressing makes it all delicious, so this is a great way of emptying out your fridge. Thin, crisp vegetables will cook much faster than others, so if you want a 10-minute dinner, use mushrooms, courgettes, mangetout, peppers, pak choi, bean sprouts and any other vegetables you like that will crisp up quickly. You can also use squash, sweet potato, carrots and aubergine, but ensure they are finely chopped or even grated before frying.

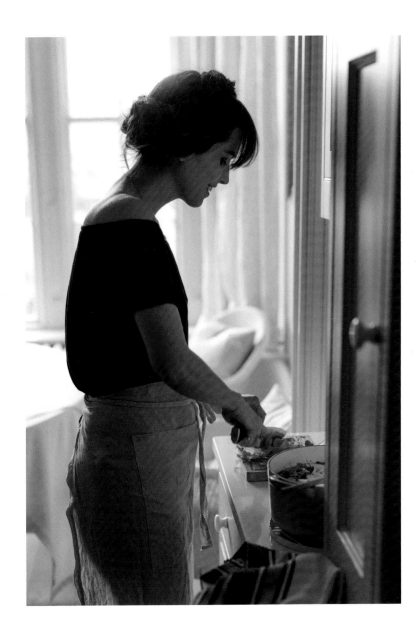

ROASTED MISO AUBERGINES WITH SESAME SEEDS

A simple aubergine can be truly transformed into a gorgeous main course. I served this at a birthday dinner party to a table of non-vegans and they all really enjoyed it. The miso adds a richness and an intense flavour, and by roasting it you get a lovely caramelised texture.

Serves 2 as a main or 4 as a side

2 aubergines

olive oil

1 tablespoon coconut or caster sugar

1 tablespoon mirin

1 tablespoon sake

1½ teaspoons miso paste

a pinch of sesame seeds, to serve

1   Slice the aubergines in half lengthways and score the white flesh in the middle in a diamond pattern, as if you were playing a game of noughts and crosses, being careful not to pierce the skin or cut the edges.

2   Heat a little olive oil in a large frying pan set over a medium-high heat. Add the aubergines, skin side down, and cook for 5 minutes. Turn over so that they are cut side down and fry for 8 minutes before putting on the lid, reducing the heat and cooking for 5 minutes more to allow them to cook through. At this point the aubergines should be very soft.

3   Make the miso glaze by whisking the sugar, mirin, sake and miso paste together.

4   Turn on the grill. If your frying pan can't go under the grill, line a baking tray with tin foil.

5   Using tongs or a fish slice, gently transfer the aubergines to the tray (if using). Brush the aubergines with the miso glaze, really pressing the sauce into the grooves.

6   Put under the grill for about 5 minutes, until the glaze is starting to bubble up. The aubergines will be piping hot, so allow them to rest for a few minutes before transferring to warmed plates and topping with a pinch of sesame seeds.

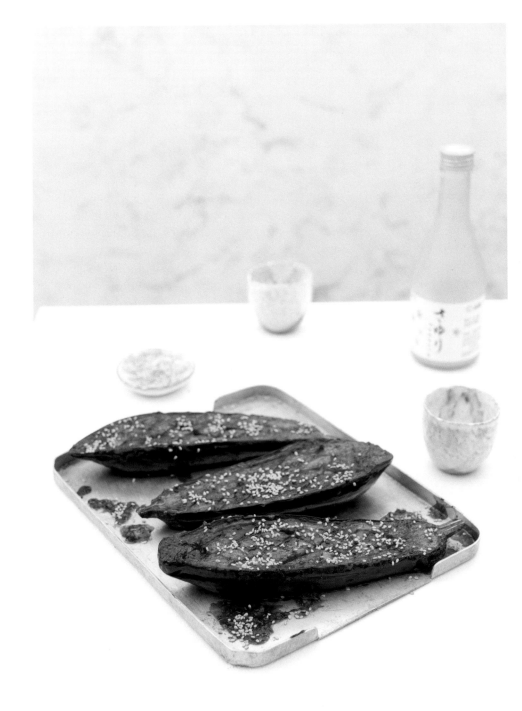

VEGAN MEATBALLS

These are a real crowd pleaser. I wasn't entirely sure what to expect the first time I made these, but I had a good feeling that they would work out and now this is one of my staple dinners.
Serves 4

FOR THE MEATBALLS:

1 tablespoon chia seeds

1 tablespoon filtered water

2 shallots, chopped

3½ oz (100g) walnuts

1 lb (50g) uncooked peeled sweet
   potato

3½ oz (100g) oyster mushrooms

½ oz (15g) nutritional yeast

pinch of salt and pepper

TO SERVE:

1 batch of tomato sauce (page 304)

courgetti (see page 116) or spaghetti

a handful of pine nuts

a handful of chopped fresh flat-leaf
   parsley

a drizzle of truffle oil or good-quality
   extra virgin olive oil

1 Preheat the oven to 350°F (180°C). Line a baking tray with non-stick baking paper.

2 First put the chia seeds and water in a small bowl and set aside for about 10 minutes to allow the seeds to gel.

3 Blend all the meatball ingredients, including the soaked chia seeds, in a food processor until a thick, chunky dough is formed. Roll into balls about the size of a ping pong ball. Put on the lined baking tray and bake in the oven for 45 minutes.

4 Meanwhile, heat the tomato sauce in a large frying pan set over a medium heat. Add the baked meatballs and simmer gently for a few minutes to bring it all together.

5 Serve in warmed shallow bowls over courgetti or spaghetti. Top with pine nuts, fresh parsley and a drizzle of truffle oil or your best extra virgin olive oil.

TIPS: If you have an extra 5 minutes, lightly fry the meatballs in some olive oil before adding them to the sauce to give them a slight crunch and a little more bite.

It's also nice to toast the pine nuts. Put them in a dry frying pan set over a medium heat and cook for a few minutes, until lightly toasted.

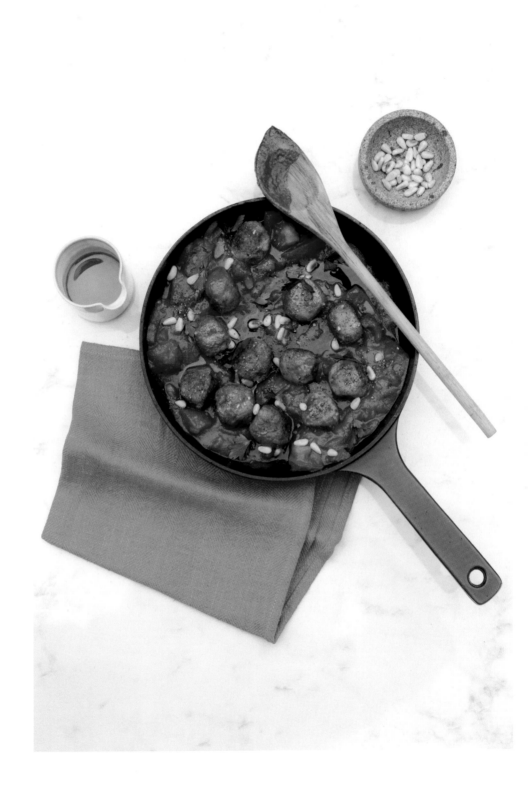

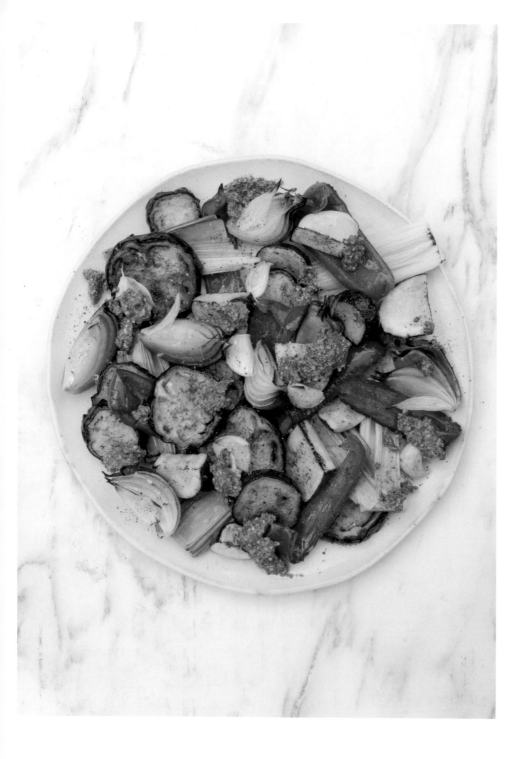

ROASTED MEDITERRANEAN VEG WITH PESTO

1 Preheat the oven to 350°F (180°C).

2 Put all the vegetables and the rosemary sprigs on a large baking tray, drizzle with olive oil, season well with salt and pepper and mix well with your hands or a spoon to coat all the veg in the oil. If the tray is too crowded, split the veg between two trays, as otherwise they will be soggy. Roast in the oven for up to 50 minutes, stirring the veg and shaking the tray halfway through.

3 When the veg come out of the oven, squeeze the garlic out of its skin – it will come out easily. Scatter the olives over and toss to combine.

4 Drizzle the pesto on top, but keep some back so that people can add extra if they like or dip bread into it.

5 Serve on warmed plates with a simple rocket salad, herby couscous or warm focaccia.

TIP: This is equally tasty cold and is perfect for eating on the go.

This is a great way to use up extra vegetables in your fridge and you can make it to suit what you have. Carrots and squash work well here, but as they are thicker root veg, give them 15 minutes of extra roasting time before adding the other ingredients. The pesto brings it all together and injects a really Mediterranean taste to it.

Serves 6

3 red onions, quartered

2 red peppers, cut into quarters

2 courgettes, halved lengthways
    and cut into chunks

2 leeks, thickly sliced

1 aubergine, cut into cubes

4 garlic cloves, unpeeled and
    squashed with the back of a
    wooden spoon

a few sprigs of fresh rosemary

olive oil

sea salt and freshly ground
    black pepper

a handful of pitted black olives
    (optional)

vegan pesto (page 239), to serve

rocket salad, herby couscous or
    focaccia, to serve

SHEPHERDLESS PIE WITH LENTILS

When I first transitioned to a plant-based diet, it was summer and light dishes felt nourishing. As I moved towards the colder months, though, I really craved comfort foods that would be warming and satisfying. This shepherdless pie ticks all the boxes.

Serves 6

1 vegan stock cube

olive oil, for frying

3½ oz (100g) button mushrooms, quartered

3 large carrots, chopped

2 medium onions, chopped

3 garlic cloves, minced

7 oz (200g) dried black or green lentils, rinsed, or 2 x 14 oz (400g) tins of green or black lentils, drained and rinsed

1 x 14 oz (400g) tin of chopped tomatoes

a handful of chopped walnuts (optional)

10½ oz (300g) frozen petit pois or peas

1 tablespoon miso paste

sea salt and freshly ground black pepper

FOR THE MASH TOPPING:

2¼ lb (1kg) potatoes, peeled and diced

1 garlic clove, minced

1 cup (250ml) unsweetened plant-based milk

1 tablespoon olive oil, plus extra for drizzling

1 tablespoon nutritional yeast (optional)

1 First dissolve the stock cube in 1 cup (250ml) of just-boiled water. Set aside.

2 Heat a little olive oil in a frying pan set over a medium heat. Add the mushrooms, carrots, onions and garlic and sauté for 8 minutes, until they are beginning to soften. Add the lentils, tinned tomatoes, walnuts (if using) and stock and simmer for 20 minutes.

3 Meanwhile, steam or boil the potatoes for about 20 minutes, until soft. Drain and place in a large bowl with the garlic, milk, olive oil and nutritional yeast (if using). Mash until smooth with a potato masher or use a hand-held blender.

4 Preheat the oven to 350°F (180°C).

5 To finish the filling, stir in the frozen peas and miso paste. Taste it at this stage to ensure you're happy with the flavour and season with salt and pepper if you think it needs it.

6 Pour the filling into a baking dish. Top with the mash and add a drizzle of olive oil.

7 Bake in the oven for 30 minutes. For the last 3 minutes, put it under the grill to crisp up the mash topping. It will be piping hot, so allow it to sit for at least 10 minutes before serving on warmed plates.

TIPS: The walnuts are optional, but they add an almost chewy texture.

If you happen to have a bottle of red wine open, adding a splash to the filling would make it even more tasty.

You can make this pie in advance or freeze it – just allow it to defrost completely before cooking in the oven for 30 minutes.

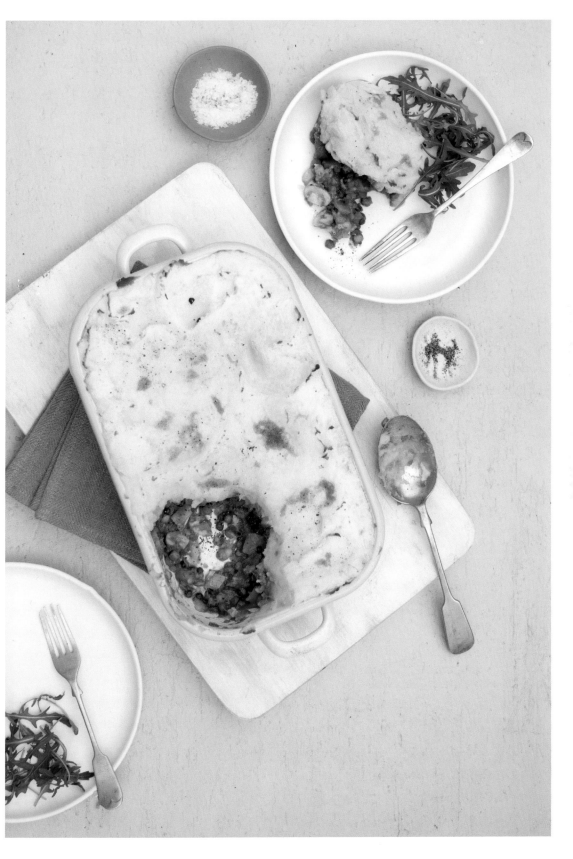

BEETROOT, CHICKPEA AND MISO BURGERS

These hearty, filling and super tasty burgers also have the appearance of rare beef mince! You can serve them in a bun but I find that almost too filling, so I usually just serve them with a spoonful of garlic mayo.

Makes 6 burgers

7 oz (200g) sweet potato

olive oil, for frying

7 oz (200g) beetroot, peeled and grated

1 small onion (approx. 2¾ oz [80g]), finely chopped

2 garlic cloves, crushed

1 x 14 oz (400g) tin of chickpeas, drained and rinsed

1½ oz (40g) walnuts, chopped

¾ oz (20g) jumbo oats

1 tablespoon tamari, soy sauce or coconut aminos

3 tablespoons ground flaxseeds

1 tablespoon nutritional yeast

1 teaspoon garlic powder

1 teaspoon miso paste

1 teaspoon fine sea salt

a pinch of freshly ground black pepper

TO SERVE:

6 burger buns, toasted (optional)

1–2 ripe avocados, peeled, stoned and sliced

1–2 ripe tomatoes, sliced

pickles

garlic mayonnaise (page 237)

1 Preheat the oven to 350°F (180°C).

2 Scrub your sweet potato clean and prick a few times with a fork so that it doesn't explode while cooking. Put on a baking tray and roast in the oven for 30 minutes, until cooked through. Set aside to cool.

3 Heat a little olive oil in a frying pan set over a medium heat. Add the beetroot, onion and garlic and lightly fry for 10 minutes, until the beetroot is cooked and the onion is starting to go transparent.

4 Combine all the remaining ingredients in a large mixing bowl, then mash until the chickpeas are broken up. You could also put all the ingredients in a food processor and pulse to combine. Add the cooked beetroot, onion and garlic and stir to combine.

5 Cut the sweet potato along the skin and the flesh should pop straight out. Discard the skin and stir the flesh into the mixture in the bowl.

6 It's best to go in with your hands at this stage to give everything a final mix. Divide the mixture in half and form each half into three burgers to make six burgers in total. Ideally you'll put these on a plate or baking tray and leave them in the fridge for at least 1 hour or, even better, overnight to allow the burgers to firm up and the flavours to combine, but you can cook them straightaway too.

7 Heat a little olive oil in a frying pan set over a medium heat. Add the burgers to the hot oil and fry for about 8 minutes on each side, until crisp and cooked through. If you're cooking them straight from the fridge allow a little more time, as they are very dense.

8 Serve with or without a toasted bun and some avocado, tomato, pickles and garlic mayonnaise.

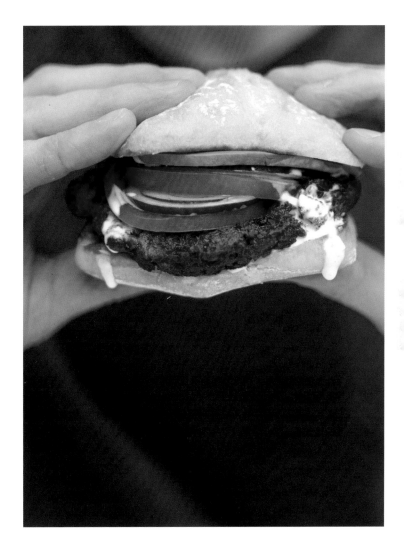

TIP: If you're cooking these on a barbecue, put an oiled square of tin foil underneath the burgers to better support them on the grill.

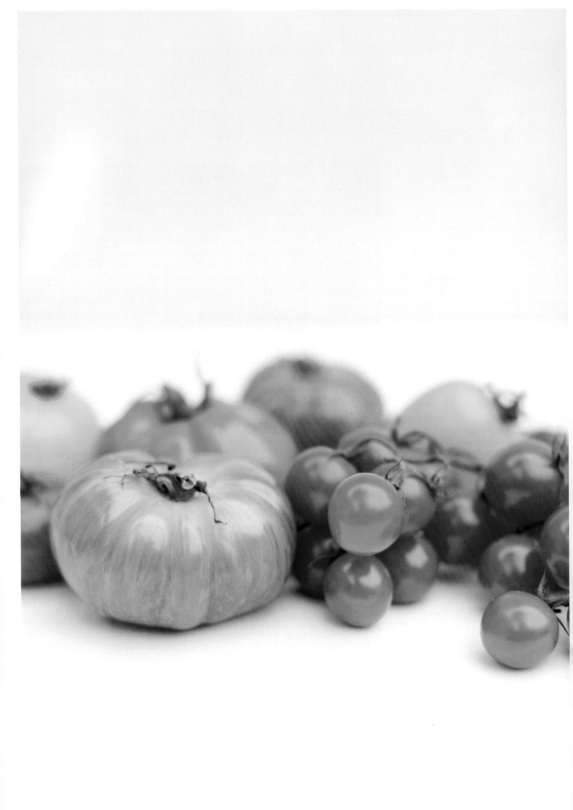

ROASTED AUBERGINE AND PESTO PASTA

1   Preheat the oven to 350°F (180°C). Line a baking tray with non-stick baking paper and brush lightly with oil.

2   Wash and dry the aubergine before slicing it thinly and placing on the prepared baking tray. Add the cherry tomatoes and garlic cloves. Roast in the oven for about 30 minutes, until the aubergines have softened.

3   Meanwhile, cook your pasta in well-salted boiling water according to the packet instructions. When it's nearly cooked and has only about 1 minute of cooking time left to go, save half a mug of the cooking water, then drain the pasta in a colander. It will continue to cook in the sauce, so be careful not to overdo it at this stage.

4   Tip the roasted aubergines and cherry tomatoes and any juices from the baking tray into the pot you cooked the pasta in. Squeeze the garlic cloves out of their skins into the pot. Mash the vegetables in the pot to break them down into a chunky sauce. Add a spoonful of the pasta cooking water, then return the pasta to the pot along with the pesto and stir to combine everything together.

5   Divide between two warmed serving dishes. Top with fresh basil and pine nuts.

TIP: It's a nice touch to toast the pine nuts. Put them in a dry frying pan set over a medium heat and cook for a few minutes, until lightly toasted. Keep an eye on them as they can quickly brown.

Although this is a simple dish, it's a fantastic quick meal with all the gorgeous Mediterranean tastes of aubergine and pesto.

Serves 2

1 aubergine

10 cherry tomatoes

2 garlic cloves, unpeeled

7 oz (200g) pasta (any kind)

1 tablespoon vegan pesto (page 239)

a few fresh basil leaves, to serve

a handful of pine nuts, to serve

CREAMY MUSHROOM PASTA WITH TAPENADE

This has all the elements of a gorgeous pasta dish. The creamy sauce and mushrooms work so well to create a delicious flavour. The slightly sour addition of the olive tapenade really balances the flavours and makes it so satisfying.

Serves 4

1 x approx. 1¾ cup (400ml) tin of coconut milk, chilled overnight

14 oz (400g) pasta (any kind)

olive oil

approx. 10 oz (280g) mushrooms (I use a mix of oyster and button mushrooms), chopped

8 shallots, finely chopped

4 garlic cloves, minced

1 large sprig of fresh thyme, leaves finely chopped

rocket salad, to serve

FOR THE TAPENADE:

2⅛ oz (60g) walnuts

20 black olives, pitted

4 tablespoons olive oil

2 tablespoons raw apple cider vinegar

sea salt and freshly ground black pepper

1 First put the tin of coconut milk in the fridge to help the creamy layer on top to separate. Ideally do this the night before.

2 Cook the pasta in boiling salted water according to the packet instructions. Reserve half a mug of the cooking water before you drain the pasta.

3 To make the tapenade, put all the ingredients in a blender or food processor and pulse to combine. I like the walnuts to maintain some of their texture, so this is more to just break them down and blend the flavours. Season to taste with salt and pepper. It will be bitter, but this gets balanced out in the finished dish by the creaminess of the mushrooms and the sweetness of the coconut. Set aside.

4 Heat a little olive oil in a large frying pan set over a medium heat. Add the mushrooms and shallots and lightly fry for 6–8 minutes, until they start to soften. Add the garlic and thyme and fry for a further minute. Add a spoonful of the pasta cooking water to the pan and simmer lightly.

5 Take the tin of coconut milk out of the fridge without shaking it. Reduce the heat under the pan to very low, then open the tin and scoop the creamy top layer into the pan, stirring to blend everything together. Season to taste with salt and pepper.

6 Drain the pasta and add it to the sauce, then quickly transfer to warmed serving plates. Add spoonfuls of the tapenade to the top of the pasta and serve in warmed shallow bowls with a simple rocket salad on the side.

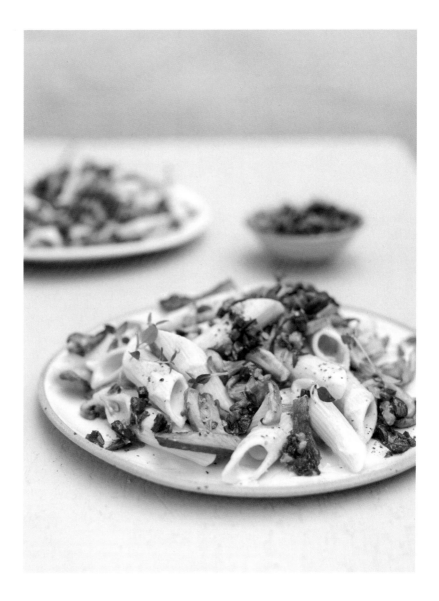

TIPS: Don't throw out the coconut water after you've scooped out the cream – save it for adding to smoothies, soups, casseroles or desserts.

The coconut will evaporate, so if you're making this in advance, do all the steps up till you add the pasta to the sauce.

You can add any leftover tapenade to dressings.

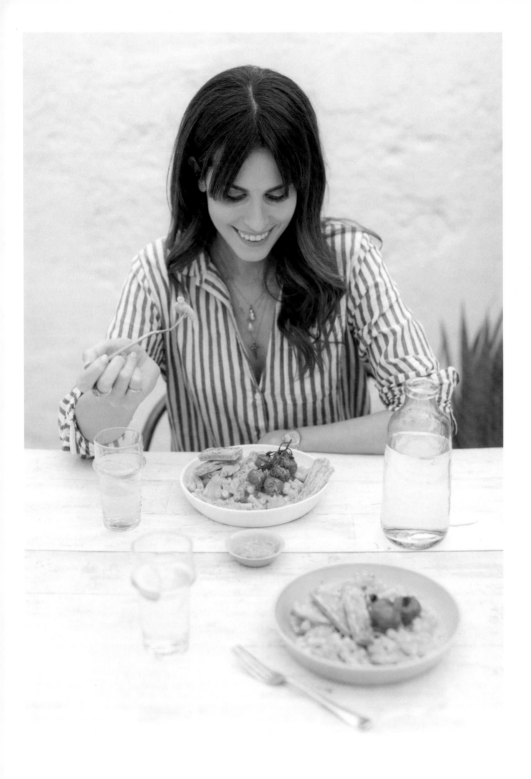

LEMONY MAC AND CHEESE WITH CHERRY TOMATOES AND CRISPY TOFU

1   Preheat the oven to 285°F (140°C).

2   Cut the butternut squash in half and scoop out the seeds. Put on a baking tray, cut side down, along with the whole unpeeled garlic cloves. Drizzle with a little olive oil and roast in the oven for about 1 hour, until soft. Set aside to cool.

3   Put the cherry tomatoes on a separate baking tray with a drizzle of olive oil and a pinch of salt and pepper. Roast in the oven along with the squash for 40 minutes. Set aside to cool.

4   While the squash and tomatoes roast, you need to press the tofu. To do this, put the tofu on a chopping board with at least four layers of kitchen paper above and below it, then wrap it up in a clean tea towel. Put a plate on top of the towel, then add a weight to the plate – a tin of beans works well. The weight will press some of the excess moisture out of the tofu, giving it a firmer texture and also enabling it to absorb more of the flavours you marinate it in. Leave it for at least 30 minutes, then unwrap the tofu and pat it dry. The amount of moisture released will surprise you!

5   Slice the tofu into strips. Mix the cornflour, bouillon and salt together in a small bowl, then dust the tofu in it.

6   Heat the vegetable oil in a large frying pan set over a medium-high heat. Add the tofu and fry for about 5 minutes, making sure it's nice and crisp before you flip it over and cook for 5 minutes on the other side. Set aside and keep warm.

(continued)

Vegan mac and cheese is one of those dishes that when you've made it once, it will become a firm favourite.

Serves 4

8¾ oz (250g) cherry tomatoes
sea salt and freshly ground
   black pepper
14 oz (400g) macaroni pasta

FOR THE CHEESE SAUCE:
1 butternut squash (approx. 2 lb
   [900g])
2 garlic cloves
½ vegan stock cube or ½ teaspoon
   vegan vegetable bouillon
1 tablespoon olive oil, plus extra
   for roasting
3 tablespoons nutritional yeast
3 tablespoons coconut milk
   (from a tin)
2 teaspoons raw apple cider vinegar
1 teaspoon mustard powder
1 teaspoon lemon zest (optional)
1 tablespoon miso paste

FOR THE CRISPY TOFU:
½ x 14 oz (400g) block of extra-firm
   tofu
2 tablespoons cornflour
½ teaspoon vegetable bouillon
½ teaspoon fine sea salt
2 tablespoons vegetable oil

7 Dissolve the stock cube or bouillon in 3⅓ fl oz (100ml) of just-boiled water. Holding the squash with a clean tea towel, scoop out the flesh into a blender. Discard the skin. Squeeze the garlic cloves out of their skins into the blender. Add the stock and all the other sauce ingredients except the miso paste. Blend thoroughly until it's a thick, creamy sauce, then stir in the miso. Taste to see if it needs a little more seasoning.

8 Cook the pasta in boiling salted water according to the packet instructions, then drain. Pour the sauce into the same pot that you cooked the pasta in. Put it on a medium heat and return the drained pasta to it. Stir together gently to combine, then add the cherry tomatoes and cook until everything is heated through.

9 Serve in warmed shallow bowls topped with the crispy tofu.

TIPS: Feel free to reduce the amount of lemon zest or leave it out altogether if you're not a fan of zesty tastes. I love it, but you can make the sauce without it and then add a little zest to a small portion to see if you like the taste. You could also add some sriracha or hot sauce to give this a little kick, or a bit more mustard also works well.

This is a very versatile sauce – try it drizzled over nachos or even roast potatoes.

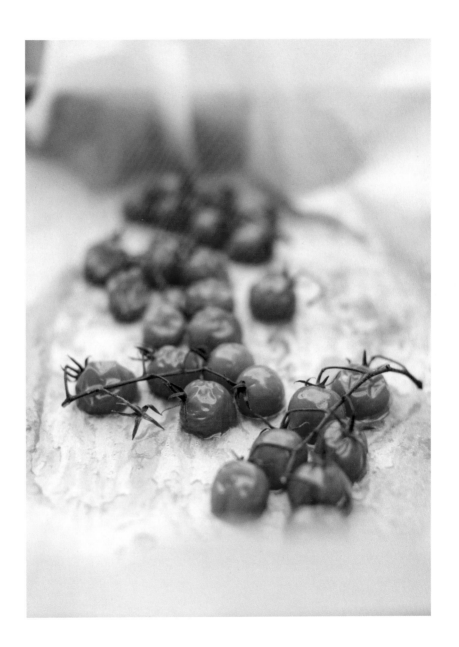

In restaurants, I have often made a meal by pairing a few side dishes together. When preparing, sides should get as much attention and care as a main course does, and all of these recipes elevate simple ingredients. They work as a fabulous addition to a main course or can be enjoyed on their own as a light bite.

SIDES

BROWN RICE WITH MISO

Years ago, when I was a student going to one of the few vegan restaurants that existed in Dublin at the time, everywhere you looked the food consisted of chunky root vegetables accompanied by a scoop of brown rice. While I thoroughly enjoyed it, nowadays I strive to inject as much flavour as possible into dishes, even side dishes, to ensure that they can all stand alone.

Serves 4

¾ lb (360g) brown rice

1 lemon, cut into wedges

sea salt and freshly ground black
    pepper

1 tablespoon miso paste

3 tablespoons olive oil

1 tablespoon tamari, soy sauce or
    coconut aminos

sesame seeds, to serve

1 Rinse the rice in a sieve until the water runs clear to remove any dust that might have settled on it. Cut the lemon in half and set one half aside, then cut the other half into wedges.

2 Bring a large pot of water to the boil. Add the lemon wedges and a good pinch of salt and pepper, then pour in the rice. Once it returns to the boil, set your timer for 25 minutes. After this time, pour the rice into a colander to drain off the water. Remove the lemon wedges and discard.

3 Return the rice to the pot and put a clean tea towel or some kitchen paper between the pot and the lid and let it sit for 5 minutes. This is the step that makes it fluffy, so don't skip it!

4 Stir the miso paste, olive oil, tamari and the juice of the remaining lemon half together, making sure you break down the miso before drizzling the dressing over the rice. Fold in the dressing with a spatula, then transfer the rice to a warmed serving bowl and scatter with sesame seeds.

TIP: Unlike white rice, which cooks by the absorption method, I think that brown rice is best cooked in lots of water. Allow 3 oz (90g) of uncooked rice per person or portion.

CHARGRILLED GREEN BEANS WITH CARAMELISED ONIONS AND GARLIC

1 Peel the onions and cut them in half, then finely slice them into half-moons. Break up the onions up as much as possible and put them in a bowl with a large pinch of salt. This helps them start to break down.

2 Heat a drizzle of olive oil in a large frying pan set over a medium heat. Add the onions and garlic and lightly fry for 10 minutes without touching them. After 10 minutes stir them around and leave them again for a further 10 minutes. Keep repeating this process, allowing them to slowly cook while you prep the rest of the food. Eventually, around the 40-minute mark, they will start sticking to the pan. Add 1 tablespoon of water, stir them around and allow them to cook for a final 10 minutes. You should have golden brown, soft, almost gooey caramelised onions at this stage. Keep them warm.

3 Put the topped and tailed green beans into a saucepan of boiling water and blanch them for 2 minutes only. Drain and plunge into a bowl of ice-cold water to halt the cooking process. Drain the water off and dry the beans thoroughly on a clean tea towel, ensuring they are as dry as possible – this is an important step.

4 Heat a little olive oil in a chargrill pan set over a high heat. When the pan is piping hot, add the green beans to the pan in batches. Be extremely careful, as any water left on the green beans will spit once it comes into contact with the hot oil, which is why you need to dry the beans so thoroughly. Grill the beans on each side for about 3 minutes without moving them to allow char marks to form.

5 Transfer to a warmed serving bowl and toss with the caramelised onions and garlic. Season with salt and pepper. There should still be enough oil on the onions to coat them, but drizzle on a tiny bit more if required. These can be served warm or cold.

Making caramelised onions is a bit time-consuming, but it's so worth it. If you have space in your frying pan, make a double batch so that you will be able to quickly recreate the dish with the pre-prepared onion. Extras can be stored in the fridge and used as sandwich and burger toppings.

Serves 4

2 large onions (approx. 1 lb [500g])

4 garlic cloves, thinly sliced

sea salt and freshly ground
    black pepper

olive oil, for frying

approx. 1 lb (500g) green beans,
    topped and tailed

LEMONY QUINOA WITH HERBS AND HAZELNUTS

This light, fluffy quinoa is the perfect accompaniment to curries or casseroles.

Serves 4

7 oz (200g) quinoa

1 teaspoon coconut oil

approx. 1¾ cup (400ml) filtered water, plus extra for soaking

1½ oz (40g) toasted hazelnuts, chopped

FOR THE DRESSING:

1 tablespoon finely chopped fresh flat-leaf parsley

1 sprig of fresh thyme, leaves stripped and finely chopped

1 sprig of fresh rosemary, leaves stripped and finely chopped

1 garlic clove, crushed

1 tablespoon olive oil

zest and juice of 1 lemon

1   Soak the quinoa in a bowl of filtered water for 15 minutes while you prep all the other ingredients. Drain it in a sieve and rinse it under the tap. Shake it thoroughly to remove as much of the water as possible.

2   Put the coconut oil into whatever pan you will be cooking the quinoa in – you need one that has a lid – and allow to melt over a medium-high heat. When the oil is nearly smoking, add the quinoa and stir it around. The water will evaporate and you will start to hear a popping sound. Keep an eye on it at this stage, as it can burn easily. If you feel it's too hot, remove the pan from the heat straight away and shake the pan to distribute heat and prevent the quinoa burning.

3   After about 2 minutes, when it's becoming lightly golden, add the filtered water and reduce the heat to medium-low. Cover the pan with a lid and simmer for 15–20 minutes, until all the water has evaporated and the quinoa is cooked. Turn off the heat, then put a clean tea towel or a piece of kitchen paper between the pot and the lid and leave it to sit for 5 minutes.

4   While your quinoa is cooking, combine all the herbs with the garlic, olive oil and the lemon juice and lemon zest.

5   While the quinoa is still warm, drizzle it with the dressing and toss together with a fork to fluff up the quinoa. Transfer to a warmed serving dish and top with the chopped toasted hazelnuts.

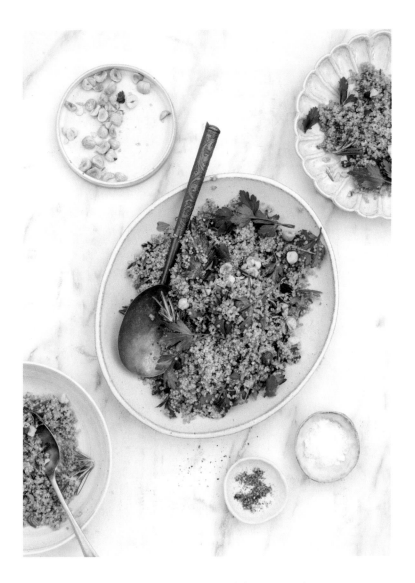

TIPS: You can buy hazelnuts that have already been toasted or use a damp clean tea towel to rub off the loose skins after toasting them on a dry frying pan for a few minutes.

For meal prepping, allow the quinoa to cool completely and store it in an airtight container in your fridge for up to three days.

GARLICKY SAUTÉED KALE WITH ALMONDS

If I'm honest, kale is not the nicest vegetable on its own. However, if it's prepared with a little bit of care, it can be transformed into something dinner party-worthy.

Serves 4

7 oz (200g) kale

a handful of flaked almonds

3 garlic cloves, thinly sliced

½ teaspoon chilli flakes

olive oil

Maldon sea salt and freshly ground
   black pepper

1   Cut out the thick stems of the kale and discard, then tear the leaves into shreds to make it easier to eat. Rinse under cold water and shake off any excess or spin it in a salad spinner. You want it to be as dry as possible.

2   Put a dry frying pan over a medium heat. Add the flaked almonds and toast, shaking the pan occasionally, until they're golden. Tip out of the pan and set aside.

3   Heat a drizzle of olive oil in the same pan, still set over a medium heat. Add the garlic and chilli flakes and sauté for 1 minute, stirring regularly to ensure the garlic doesn't burn.

4   Add a layer of kale and use kitchen tongs to toss it in the garlic and oil. Allow it to cook for about 1 minute on each side before transferring it to a hot serving dish and getting the next layer of kale into the pan. It's amazing how much it wilts!

5   Scatter the toasted flaked almonds on top and add a pinch of crushed sea salt and fresh black pepper before serving.

TIP: Kale cools extremely quickly, so make sure you have a plate warming to put it on to serve straight away.

ROASTED AUBERGINES WITH MISO CREAM AND PINE NUTS

1 Put the cashews in a bowl, cover with cold filtered water and soak for at least 8 hours or ideally overnight. Drain and rinse, then pat them dry thoroughly with a clean tea towel or kitchen paper. (See the note on page 30 on soaking nuts.)

2 Put the aubergine wedges in a colander set over a bowl and sprinkle with a good pinch of fine sea salt while you prep the rest of the ingredients. After about 20 minutes, water will have drained off them and they will have beads of water on them. This will make them taste much lighter and is worth the extra effort.

3 Meanwhile, make the dressing by putting the soaked cashews in a high-powered blender and processing until they are silky smooth. Add the lemon juice, garlic powder, agave syrup and half of the miso paste and pulse to combine. Drizzle in the water and blend until you get the texture you want. Taste it at this stage – if you want it to be richer, add the rest of the miso paste. Set aside.

4 Put a dry frying pan over a medium heat. Add the pine nuts and cook for a few minutes, until lightly toasted. Tip out onto a plate.

5 Preheat the oven to 400°F (200°C). Generously oil a baking tray.

6 Pat the aubergines with kitchen paper to dry them and to remove the salt. Put on the oiled tray and roast in the oven for about 25 minutes, checking at the 20-minute mark to shuffle them around and turn the tray around in the oven if you find that the ones at the back are getting the most heat and are cooking unevenly.

7 Allow the wedges to cool slightly before serving on warmed plates with a drizzle of dressing and the pine nuts scattered on top.

Aubergines take on a richness that's unparalelled when they are given a little bit of time and attention. The addition of the miso cream here dresses them up and these will quickly disappear wherever they are served.

Serves 4

3 medium aubergines, cut into
    wedges
fine sea salt or Himalayan pink salt
olive oil, for greasing
a handful of pine nuts

FOR THE MISO CREAM:
approx. 4½ oz (125g) cashew nuts
1 tablespoon lemon juice
1 teaspoon garlic powder
1 teaspoon agave syrup
1 tablespoon miso paste
4¼ fl oz (125ml) filtered water

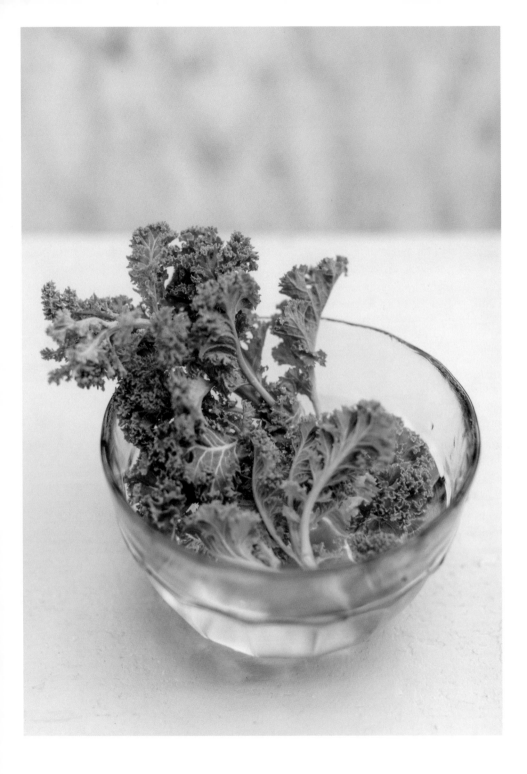

KALE WITH ROASTED CHICKPEAS AND TAHINI DRESSING

1   Preheat the oven to 300°F (150°C).

2   You want the chickpeas to get as crisp as possible, so pat them dry with a clean tea towel or kitchen paper.

3   Drizzle a little olive oil into a baking tray. Pour the chickpeas into the tray and add the tamari and garlic powder. Use your hands or a spoon to toss the chickpeas, making sure they're all coated in the oil, tamari and garlic. Roast on the bottom rack of the oven for about 40 minutes, shaking the tray halfway through, until the chickpeas are crisp.

4   Meanwhile, strip the kale leaves from the thick rib, then shred the leaves and put in a large mixing bowl. Pour the tahini dressing over the kale and use your hands to massage it in.

5   When the chickpeas are ready, allow them to cool for a few minutes before tossing them through the kale.

TIP: Some sliced avocado works really well with this dish.

Kale has a thick cell wall, but the acids in the vinegar or lemon juice will help to break it down and soften the kale, which makes it nicer to eat, but you have to massage it in really well. Allow at least 10 minutes for this.

Serves 4

1 x 14 oz (400g) tin of chickpeas,
    drained and rinsed
olive oil, for roasting
1 tablespoon tamari, soy sauce or
    coconut aminos
½ teaspoon garlic powder
3½ oz (100g) kale
1 batch of tahini dressing (page 232)

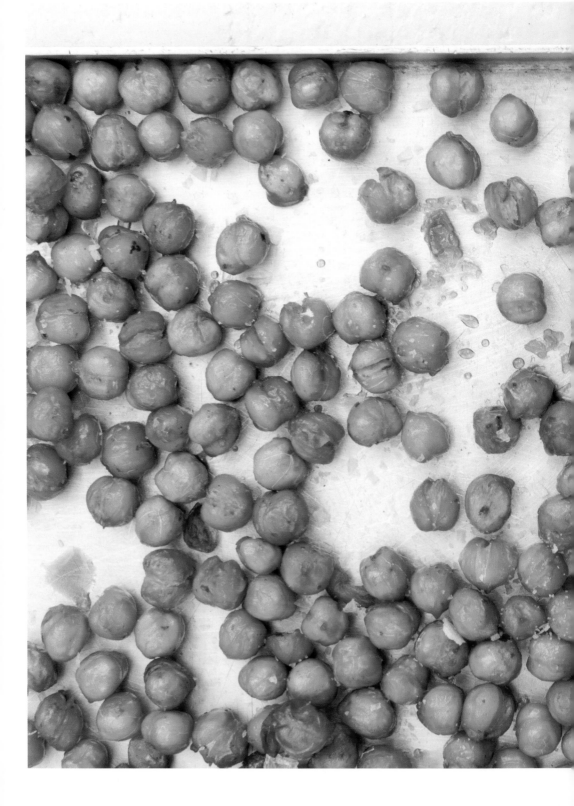

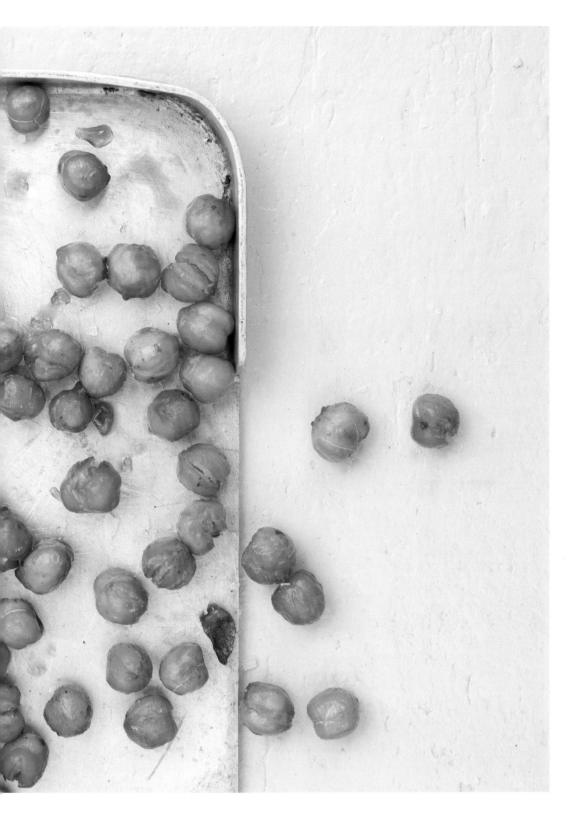

BROCCOLI AND CAULIFLOWER CHEESE

Cauliflower cheese is one of those delicious comfort foods. The broccoli here adds a little colour and a different texture too.

Serves 4

1 head of broccoli, cut into florets
    (approx. 14 oz [400g])
½ head of cauliflower, cut into florets
    (approx. 10½ oz [300g])
2 garlic cloves, crushed
1 tablespoon olive oil
1 teaspoon onion powder

FOR THE SAUCE:

2 tablespoons olive oil
4 garlic cloves, crushed
3 tablespoons cornflour
scant 2 cup (450ml) unsweetened
    plain almond milk
3 heaped tablespoons
    nutritional yeast
1 tablespoon lemon juice
1 heaped teaspoon prepared English
    mustard or mustard powder
¼ teaspoon fine sea salt
¼ teaspoon ground black pepper

1   Preheat the oven to 350°F (180°C).
2   Blanch the broccoli and cauliflower in boiling salted water for 2 minutes before straining in a colander. Put them in the baking dish that you will cook them in. Add the garlic, oil and onion powder and mix well together to combine.
3   To make the sauce, heat the oil in a saucepan set over a medium heat. Add the garlic and fry for 1 minute, then add the cornflour. Pour in a little almond milk and whisk to form a paste, then slowly pour in the rest of the milk, whisking until you have a creamy sauce.
4   Use a hand-held blender to purée it or transfer to a blender to make sure it's silky smooth. Add the nutritional yeast, lemon juice, mustard or mustard powder, salt and pepper. Pour the sauce over the broccoli and cauliflower.
5   Bake in the oven for 25–30 minutes, until the vegetables are soft and the sauce is bubbling. For a slightly smoky, charred taste, put it under the grill for 2–3 minutes at the very end.

TIP: You can add some vegan cheese if you have a brand you like. Put a layer of it on top at the last minute before grilling.

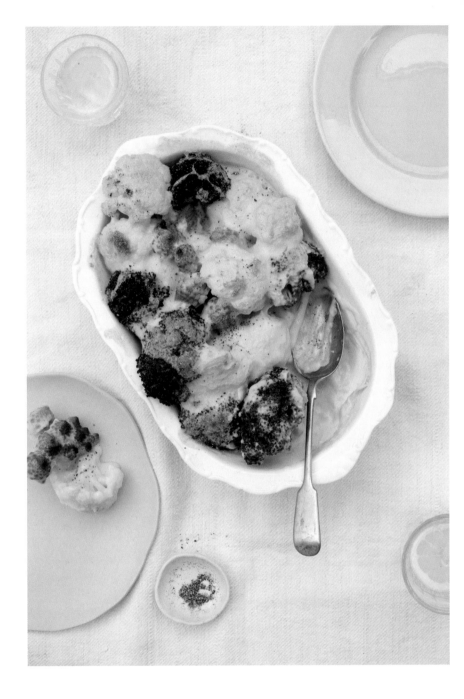

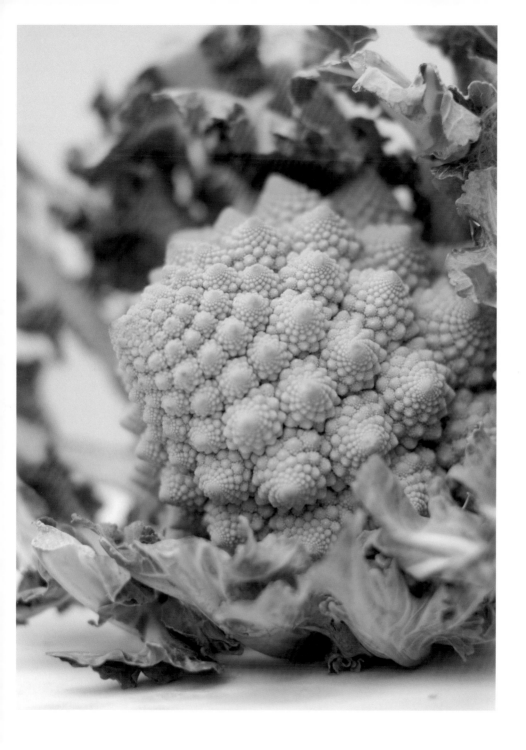

CRISPY ROASTED CAULIFLOWER WITH CILANTRO

1 Preheat the oven to 350°F (180°C).

2 Wash the cauliflower and remove the outer leaves. Break up the cauliflower into bite-sized pieces by hand – it will crumble too much if you cut it with a knife.

3 Mix the spices and olive oil in a large bowl, then add the cauliflower. Using a spoon or your hands, toss to coat the cauliflower in the spices as evenly as possible.

4 Put on a baking tray and roast in the oven for 30 minutes, tossing the cauliflower midway through to make sure it cooks evenly and doesn't burn. Remove from the oven and season to taste with salt and pepper.

5 Transfer to a warmed serving dish and scatter some sesame seeds on top for a bit of extra texture. Scatter over some chopped fresh cilantro, add a drizzle of olive oil and serve piping hot.

TIP: This can be served hot or cold and holds well in the fridge for up to three days in an airtight container.

I first had something like this in a restaurant as a side and I couldn't get over how tasty it was. I set out to create my own version at home and was surprised at how easy it is to make cauliflower taste amazing. This is the most perfect side dish and is quick enough to make during the week. I love it with some tofu, a green salad and lots of hummus.

Serves 4

2 heads of cauliflower

1 teaspoon ground turmeric

1 teaspoon ground cumin

½ teaspoon paprika

½ teaspoon garlic powder

a drizzle of olive oil

sea salt and freshly ground
    black pepper

a pinch of sesame seeds, to serve

½ bunch of fresh cilantro, chopped

POTATO AND ONION GRATIN

In the depths of recipe testing for this book, my friends and family had most likely reached a stage where they didn't want to taste another thing. But when this was bubbling away in the oven, filling the house with the gorgeous smell of roasting onions, I brought a little bowl of it over to him. After just one bite, he looked up at me and said, 'That's really special.' I hope you'll think so too.

Serves 6

1¾ lb (800g) potatoes
   (I use Kerr's Pink)
6 shallots
1 onion
1 x approx. 1¾ cup (400ml) tin of
   coconut milk
1¼ cup (300ml) soy milk
5 garlic cloves, crushed
1 large sprig of fresh thyme
3 tablespoons nutritional yeast
1½ teaspoons mustard powder
sea salt and freshly ground
   black pepper

1   If you have a slicer setting on your food processor, you'll fly through this. Simply peel the potatoes, shallots and onion. Put the potatoes through the processor or use a mandolin or slice them very thinly. At this stage I like to put them in a colander and rinse some of the starch off them.

2   Put the shallot and onion through the processor or thinly slice them by hand.

3   Pour the coconut and soy milk into a large saucepan. Add the garlic, thyme, nutritional yeast, mustard and some salt and pepper. Bring to the boil, stirring to blend all the flavours evenly, then turn down the heat. Add the potatoes, shallots and onion and simmer for 5 minutes.

4   Carefully pour everything into a large baking dish. Cover the dish with tin foil, then bake in the oven for 1 hour. Remove the foil for the last 10 minutes and put the dish under a grill to allow the top to go crisp.

BASIL MASHED POTATOES

1   Peel the potatoes if you want a really smooth mash. I leave the skins on – it doesn't look as beautiful, but it's quicker! Steam or boil the potatoes with the whole garlic clove for about 20 minutes, until soft.

2   Discard the garlic, then transfer the potatoes to a blender or mash them in the pot by hand. Add the minced garlic, milk, nutritional yeast and olive oil and blend or mash together. If you're using a blender, don't over-blend and use the plunger to ensure all the ingredients are mixed together.
Fold in the basil by hand and season to taste with salt and pepper.

3   Transfer the mashed potatoes into a warmed serving bowl. Drizzle with a little olive oil and garnish with the remaining basil leaves.

TIP: I'm personally not a fan of vegan butters, but they can be used in place of the olive oil if you like.

Vegan mashed potatoes are a bit of a revelation. This is creamy, comforting and delicious – all the things you would associate with a traditional mash.

Serves 4

1⅓ lb (600g) potatoes, diced

1 garlic clove, left whole

1 garlic clove, minced

1 cup (250ml) unsweetened plant-based milk

1 tablespoon nutritional yeast

1 tablespoon olive oil, plus extra for drizzling

½ oz (15g) fresh basil, chopped (save some of the leaves for garnish)

sea salt and freshly ground black pepper

ROASTED PEPPERS WITH CHERRY TOMATOES, CAPERS AND OLIVES

This is a gorgeous side that will brighten up any plate. It's very simple and only requires a few minutes of prep time. My mum makes this all the time without the olives and capers. I adore the salty, rich flavour that they bring to it, so this is my take on her speciality.

Serves 4

4 red peppers, sliced

8 cherry tomatoes

8 garlic cloves, peeled

12–15 black olives, pitted and halved

1 tablespoon olive oil, plus extra
    for drizzling

1 tablespoon capers

a few fresh basil leaves

1 Preheat the oven to 350°F (180°C).

2 Cut the peppers in half vertically and remove the core and seeds. Put the halves on a baking tray, cut side up. Put one cherry tomato and one peeled garlic clove into each half.

3 Purée the black olives, olive oil and capers in a small bowl. Add a teaspoon of this mix to each of the peppers. Drizzle olive oil over everything, then roast in the oven for 45 minutes.

4 Shred a few fresh basil leaves on top before serving on warmed plates.

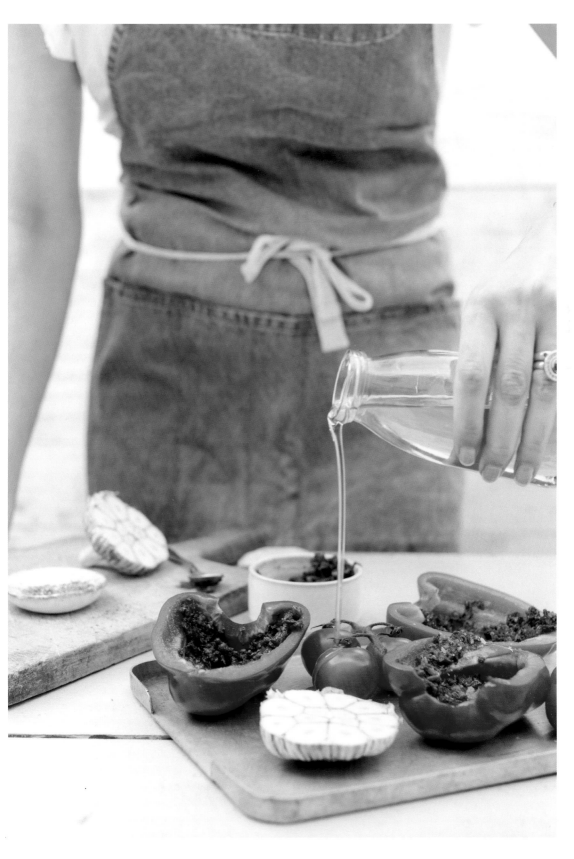

ROSEMARY AND MAPLE ROASTED CARROTS

Simple carrots become something really special here. Steaming them first and allowing some of the moisture to evaporate is key, as this gives them a head start in the cooking and also allows them to crisp up a little quicker.

Serves 4

2¼ lb (1kg) carrots

1 tablespoon olive oil

1 tablespoon maple syrup

4 sprigs of fresh rosemary, leaves stripped

1   Preheat the oven to 350°F (180°C).

2   Scrub the carrots really well. I like to leave the skin on, but you can peel them if you prefer. Cut them in half lengthways. Put the carrots on to steam for 5 minutes. Leave them to stand for a minute or so to allow some of the moisture to evaporate.

3   Mix the olive oil, maple syrup and rosemary in the bottom of the tray that you will roast the carrots in. Add the carrots and toss them in the oil. Spread them out in the tray with as much space as possible between them so that they can get enough heat.

4   Roast in the oven for up to 30 minutes, shaking the pan halfway though to ensure they cook evenly.

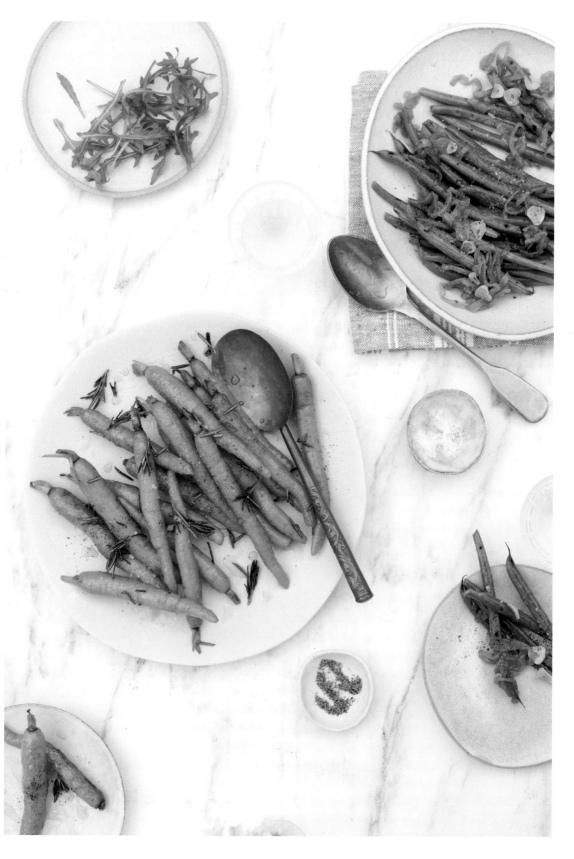

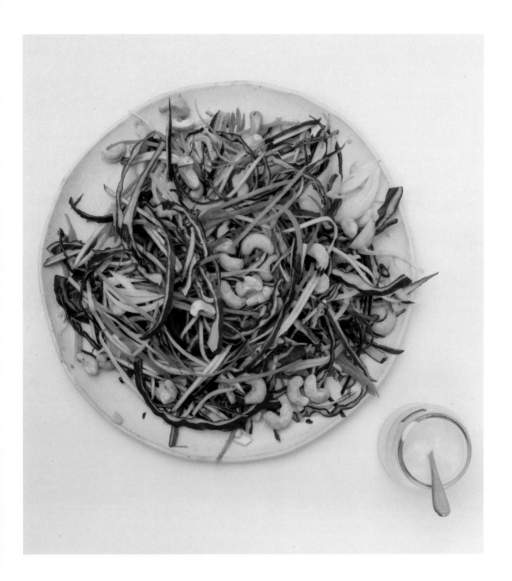

CASHEW AND CABBAGE SLAW

1   Put all the vegetables in a large bowl. Stir in the mayo until everything is well combined. Season to taste with salt and pepper, then top with toasted cashew nuts.

2   Stored in an airtight container in the fridge, this will keep for up to three days.

This is a great way of making raw cabbage and carrots actually taste delicious! They key ingredient that brings it all together is the vegan mayonnaise.

Serves 4

2 carrots, grated

1 courgette, grated

1 onion, finely diced

½ head of red cabbage, grated

1 batch of vegan mayo (page 236)

sea salt and freshly ground
   black pepper

a handful of toasted cashew nuts

CREAMY SWEET POTATO MASH

Sweet potato mash brings a totally different element to a meal.

Serves 4

1⅓ lb (600g) sweet potatoes

2 garlic cloves, minced

½ fresh red chilli, deseeded and
    chopped (optional)

1 tablespoon olive oil

sea salt and freshly ground
    black pepper

approx. 4–5 fl oz (100–200ml)
    unsweetened plant-based milk

a pinch of paprika (optional)

1   Preheat the oven to 300°F (150°C).

2   Scrub your potatoes clean and prick each one a few times with a fork so they don't explode while cooking. Put on a baking tray and roast in the oven for about an hour, until cooked through.

3   Remove from the oven and give them a few minutes to allow them to cool down, then slice them in half. Use a clean tea towel to hold them; they should easily pop out of their skins or you can scoop out the flesh.

4   Sweet potatoes, unlike their white counterparts, mash really easily. Simply transfer them to a bowl with the garlic, chilli (if using), olive oil, some salt and pepper and 3⅓ fl oz (100ml) of the milk and mash everything together. Judge the consistency at this stage and see if you think it needs more milk. You might not need to use it all.

5   Transfer to a warmed serving dish. You can top this with a pinch of paprika if you want some warmth.

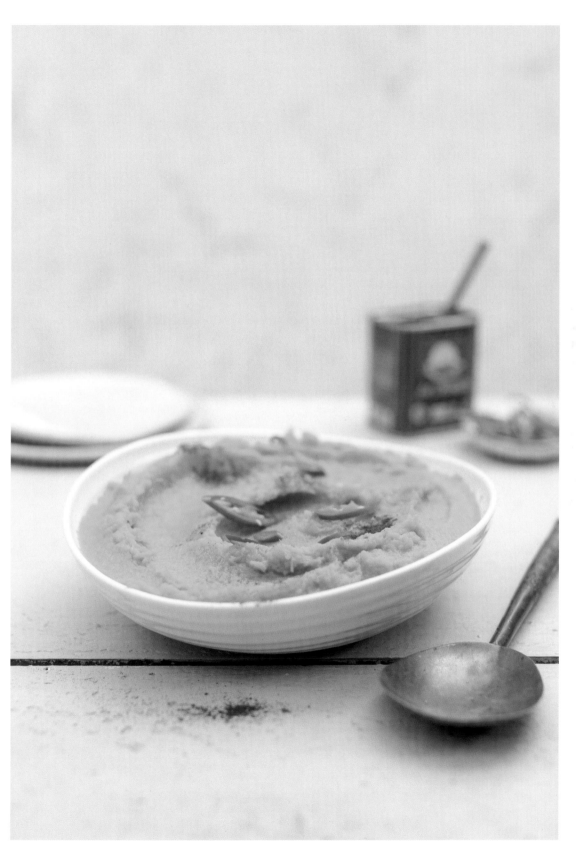

SWEET POTATO WEDGES WITH CASHEW CHEESE

When I first transitioned to a vegan diet I think I must have eaten sweet potato wedges or fries at least twice a week for a year. As a result, I got pretty good at cooking them. Keeping them chunky means they become the perfect vessel to dip into a delicious sauce, and this cashew cheese dip complements their sweetness perfectly.

Serves 4

1¾ lb (800g) sweet potatoes,
   scrubbed and dried
2 tablespoons olive oil
2–3 sprigs of fresh thyme, leaves
   stripped, or 1 teaspoon dried thyme
sea salt and freshly ground
   black pepper
a pinch of paprika (optional)
cashew cheese (page 305), to serve

1 Preheat the oven to 350°F (180°C).

2 Cut the sweet potatoes into wedges, then slice the wedges in half, then quarters and cut once again if they are still too big. Put them in a bowl and coat them in the olive oil, thyme and some pepper. Put them on a baking tray, ensuring they all have some space around them and are not overcrowded or they will steam, not roast. Bake in the oven for at least 40 minutes, tossing halfway though, until cooked through and crisp.

3 Put the wedges on a warmed serving dish and season with salt. Top with a dusting of paprika if you like a little heat. Put the cashew cheese in a smaller serving dish and set it in the centre of the wedges for dipping.

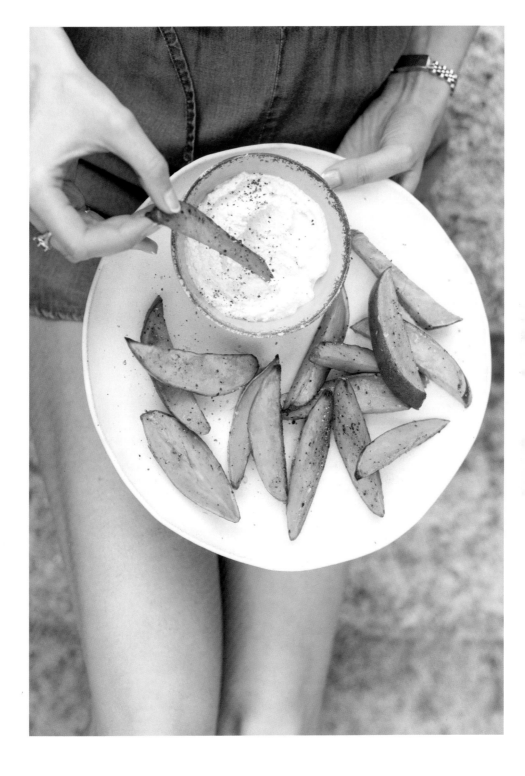

THE BEST ROAST POTATOES WITH ROASTED GARLIC SAUCE

There are whole books written on roast potatoes and countless theories, methods and ideas on what makes the perfect roast potato. Perfection is a hard thing to strive for, but I think these come very close. I remember one of my friends referring to 'the polite potato', aka a lone spud that everyone wants but is being too polite to take. That won't happen with these! But enough talk. Here's how to make them.

Serves 6

approx. 2¼ lb (1kg) Maris Piper
   potatoes

1 garlic clove, peeled

1 tablespoon olive oil

FOR THE GARLIC SAUCE:

3½ oz (100g) cashews

1 head of garlic

2 teaspoons olive oil

4¼ fl oz (125ml) filtered water

1 tablespoon nutritional yeast

1 tablespoon olive oil

1 teaspoon lemon juice

1   Put the cashews in a bowl, cover with filtered water and soak for at least 8 hours or ideally overnight. Drain and rinse, then pat them dry thoroughly with a clean tea towel or kitchen paper. (See the note on page 30 on soaking nuts.)

2   Personally I like the skins left on – plus it makes for a much faster preparation time – but do whatever you like best, peeled or unpeeled. Chop the potatoes into a semi-uniform size to ensure they cook evenly – about the size of a golf ball is a good guide. Put in a pot with the whole garlic clove, cover with plenty of cold water and bring to the boil, then reduce the heat and cook or 20 minutes, until tender. Drain them in a colander and allow them to sit for at least 2 minutes. The more moisture that's removed, the crispier they'll get.

3   Preheat the oven to 400°F (200°C).

4   Put the drained potatoes in a large roasting tin. Pour over the tablespoon of olive oil and shake the potatoes in the tin to bash them up a bit and coat them with oil. This creates lots of little crispy clusters.

5   Remove the papery outer layer of skin from the head of garlic, leaving the head itself intact with all the cloves still connected. Trim about ¼" (5mm) off the top of the head of garlic to expose the tops of the cloves. Put the garlic on a large piece of foil, then drizzle the 2 teaspoons of olive oil over the top and tightly seal up the foil.

6   Put the foil parcel in the corner of the roasting tin, then cook in the oven for 40 minutes. Halfway through the cooking time, take the tin out of the oven, give it a shake and turn the potatoes, ensuring they get crisp on all sides. Return to the oven for about 15 minutes more, until they look crisp.

7 Carefully open up the foil parcel of garlic, being careful of any escaping steam. Squeeze the garlic out of its skins into a small bowl.

8 Blend the soaked and drained cashews in a high-powered blender until they are silky smooth. Add all the other ingredients, including the roasted garlic, and blend well. Serve the garlic sauce on the side or pour it over your roasted potatoes.

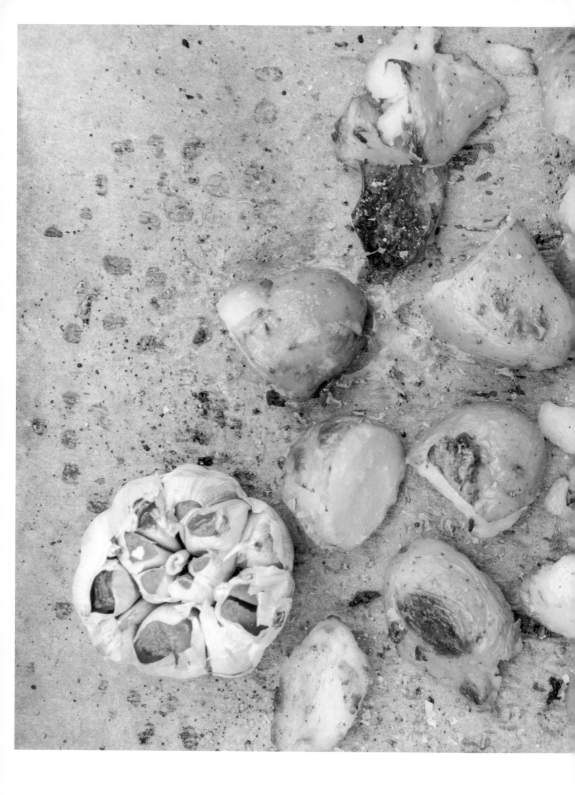

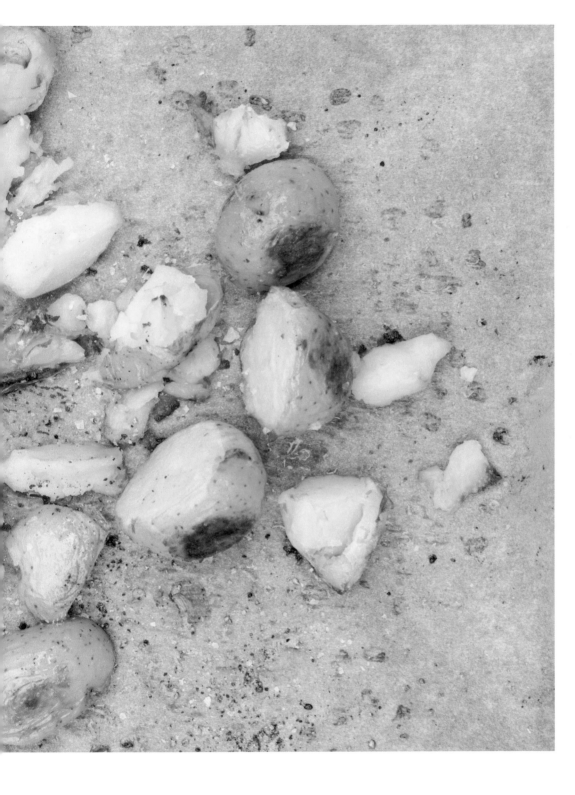

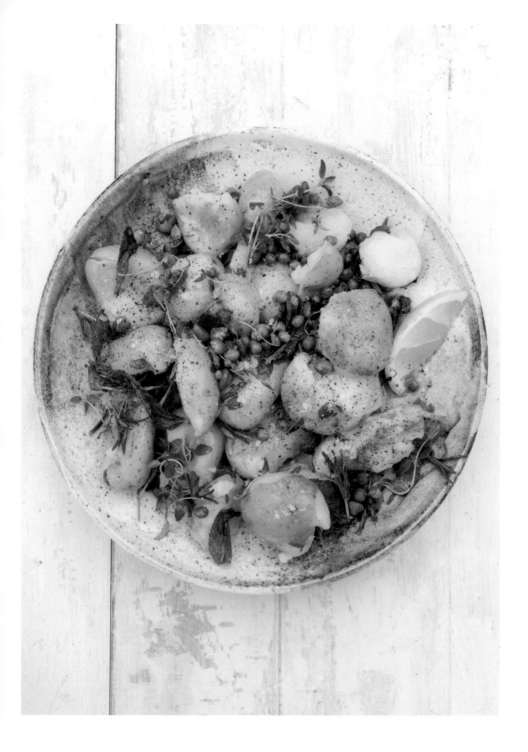

CRUSHED NEW POTATOES WITH CAPERS

1 Leave the skins on the potatoes and scrub them well. Set them on to steam above a pot of boiling water until cooked through and tender – roughly 20 minutes depending on their size. Test this by sticking a skewer or fork into them. Leave them to steam dry for approximately 5 minutes.

2 Meanwhile, leave ¾ oz (20g) of the fresh mint whole. Finely shred the leaves of the remaining ⅓ oz (10g). Combine the garlic, capers, herbs and olive oil in a large mixing bowl. Using the back of a fork, crush some of the capers to release their flavour. Set aside to infuse the oil.

3 Before you transfer the potatoes to the mixing bowl, remove the whole mint sprigs and discard them. Crush the potatoes lightly with a potato masher and toss them gently in the oil. Season with salt and pepper and a squeeze of lemon.

4 This is best served warm, not piping hot, so allow it to cool a little while you prepare the rest of your meal.

New potatoes steamed and served simply are delicious, but if you want to dress them up a little, this is a lovely way to do it.

Serves 4

approx. 2¼ lb (1kg) new potatoes

1 oz (30g) fresh mint

4 garlic cloves, crushed

approx. 2 oz (60g) caper berries, stems removed and cut in half if big, or approx. 2 oz (60g) regular capers, rinsed and left whole

⅓ oz (10g) sprigs of fresh thyme, leaves stripped

⅓ oz (10g) sprigs of fresh rosemary, leaves stripped

2½ fl oz (75ml) olive oil

sea salt and freshly ground black pepper

1 lemon wedge

Vegan desserts are a revelation. If you're looking for something creamy, beautiful and incredibly tasty, I've got you covered! It amazes me how few vegan dessert options there are in restaurants bar a bowl of berries or some plain fruit. From cheesecakes to brownies to fudge there are so many incredible recipes here that will bring the wow factor to any dinner party or hit the spot if you just want a bit of comfort food.

DESSERTS

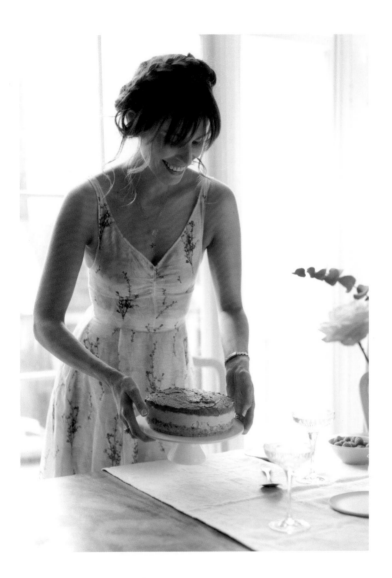

RASPBERRY AND LEMON LAYERED CHEESECAKE

1 Put the cashews for the filling in two separate bowls – the 10½ oz (300g) for the lemon layer in one bowl and the approx. 2⅔ oz (75g) for the berry layer in another bowl – cover with filtered water and soak for at least 8 hours, or ideally overnight. Drain and rinse, still keeping them separate, then pat them dry thoroughly with a clean tea towel or kitchen paper. (See the note on page 30 on soaking nuts.)

2 Line a 9" (23cm) springform cake tin with non-stick baking paper.

3 Begin with the base. Blitz the cashews and the macadamias in a food processor until a fine flour-like texture is formed. Add the desiccated coconut, dates and maple syrup and continue to process until the mixture sticks together and forms a thick dough-like consistency. Press this evenly onto the base of the lined cake tin, pushing it down firmly to make sure there are no gaps. I use the base of a glass to press it down. Put it in the freezer to set for at least 15 minutes.

4 Meanwhile, to make the lemon layer, put the 10½ oz (300g) of soaked cashews in a high-powered blender and process them for 1 minute, until smooth. Add the lemon juice, maple syrup, coconut oil and vanilla extract and continue to process for about 1 minute, until it's thick and creamy. Fold through the lemon zest. Pour the filling over the base and return to the freezer for at least 15 minutes.

5 To make the berry layer, put the 2⅔ oz (75g) of soaked cashews in a high-powered blender with the raspberries, dates and lemon juice and process until smooth. I like this to be quite sharp, but if after tasting you would like it to be sweeter, just add another date or two. Pour this on top of the lemon layer and put in the freezer to set for at least 2 hours.

(continued)

When I first made a vegan cheesecake I couldn't get over the creamy texture and how rich and satisfying it was, not to mention that the next day I didn't feel bloated like I used to when I had cream or milk. This cake takes a while to make, but it's definitely worth it. It's so beautiful, so it's definitely one to take a photo of – when you get to the end!

Serves 12

FOR THE BASE:

5¼ oz (150g) cashew nuts

5¼ oz (150g) macadamia nuts

3 oz (80g) desiccated coconut

3 oz (75g) Medjool dates, pitted

2 fl oz (60ml) maple syrup

FOR THE LEMON LAYER:

10½ oz (300g) cashew nuts

4¼ fl oz (125ml) lemon juice

4¼ fl oz (125ml) maple syrup

80ml melted coconut oil

½ teaspoon vanilla extract

1 tablespoon lemon zest

FOR THE RASPBERRY LAYER:

2⅔ oz (75g) cashew nuts

3½ oz (100g) fresh or frozen raspberries, plus extra fresh berries to decorate

2⅔ oz (75g) Medjool dates, pitted

2 tablespoons lemon juice

6 Remove the cake from the freezer and let it thaw for 30 minutes before serving. Top with fresh raspberries if you like. This will keep in the fridge for up to two weeks or for up to two months in the freezer.

MINI CARROT CAKES WITH LEMON COCONUT CREAM

There is something very wholesome-tasting about this cake, even though it's totally delicious. Carrot cake is famous for its thick, creamy icing and the coconut cream will really amaze you if you haven't made it before. I love the addition of mint – it cuts through the sweetness and balances it out.

Makes 12 mini cakes

1¼ cup (300ml) unsweetened soy milk

2 teaspoons raw apple cider vinegar

1 tablespoon ground chia seeds or flaxseeds

3 tablespoons filtered water

6⅓ oz (180g) wholemeal spelt flour

approx. 4½ oz (125g) coconut flour

1 teaspoon baking powder

1 teaspoon baking soda

2 teaspoons ground cinnamon

1 teaspoon ground ginger

½ teaspoon ground allspice or nutmeg

½ teaspoon fine sea salt

7 oz (200g) dark soft brown sugar or coconut sugar

2 tablespoons coconut oil, at room temperature, plus extra melted oil for greasing

2 teaspoons vanilla extract

5 oz (140g) carrots, grated

4¼ oz (120g) apple sauce (see recipe below)

FOR THE APPLE SAUCE:

2 medium apples (any kind), peeled, cored and chopped

6¾ fl oz (200ml) filtered water

1 tablespoon dark soft brown sugar

1 tablespoon lemon juice

¼ teaspoon ground cinnamon or ground ginger

FOR THE LEMON COCONUT CREAM:

1 batch of vanilla coconut cream (page 309)

zest of 1 lemon

TO DECORATE (OPTIONAL):

fresh mint leaves

coconut flakes

(continued)

1   To make the apple sauce, put all the ingredients in a saucepan and bring to the boil. Reduce the heat and simmer for about 15 minutes, until the apples are soft, but they might need a little longer. Purée with a hand-held blender and set aside to cool. Measure out the 5 oz (140g) of apple sauce that you'll need for the cake and store the rest in an airtight container in the fridge.

2   Preheat the oven to 350°F (170°C). I have a silicone cupcake mould, but I still brush a little melted coconut oil on the inside of each cup to make sure the cakes don't stick. If you don't have a silicone mould, you can use two 7" (18cm) cake tins and grease those with coconut oil.

3   To make the cake batter, mix together the soy milk and apple cider vinegar and set aside for about 10 minutes to let the vinegar curdle the soy milk, like buttermilk.

4   Make a chia or flax 'egg' by mixing the chia or flaxseeds and water together in a small bowl. Put in the fridge for about 10 minutes to allow it to gel.

5   Sieve the spelt flour, coconut flour, baking powder, baking soda, cinnamon, ginger, allspice or nutmeg and salt into a medium-sized bowl and stir to combine.

6   In a separate large bowl, use an electric mixer to beat together the brown sugar, coconut oil and vanilla extract until light and fluffy. Add the soy milk and vinegar mixture and the 'egg' and mix again until well combined. Fold in the dry ingredients, then fold in the grated carrots and apple sauce. It will be a thick, chunky batter.

(continued)

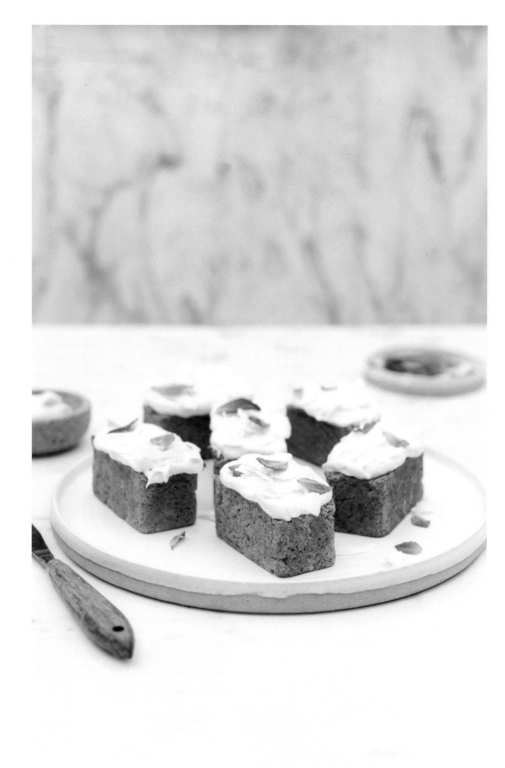

7   Spoon the batter into the cake moulds, making sure it spreads out evenly. Tap the tray on the counter to release any air bubbles. Bake in the oven for about 18 minutes, until a skewer inserted into the centre comes out clean. If you're using two larger tins, bake for 20–25 minutes.

8   Meanwhile, make the coconut cream as per the recipe on page 309 but whisk in the lemon zest along with the sweetener and vanilla.

9   Allow the cakes to cool completely on a wire rack, then pipe or spread the lemon coconut cream on top. Decorate with fresh mint leaves and coconut flakes (if using). Store the cakes in the fridge until serving to keep the coconut cream firm.

TIP: If you don't want to make your own apple sauce, buy a few jars in the baby food section!

DINNER PARTY CHOCOLATE CAKE

1   Put the cashews in a bowl, cover with filtered water and soak for at least 8 hours or ideally overnight. Drain and rinse, then pat them dry thoroughly with a clean tea towel or kitchen paper. (See the note on page 30 on soaking nuts.)

2   If your dates seem a little hard or you're using date pieces, put them in a bowl, cover with just-boiled water and soak for 10 minutes, then drain.

3   Brush a thin layer of melted coconut oil over the base and sides of a 6" (15cm) springform tin.

4   Make the base by blending the dates, walnuts, desiccated coconut and cacao powder in a food processor until well combined. Press this evenly onto the base of the greased cake tin, pushing it down firmly to make sure there are no gaps. I use the base of a glass to press it down. Put it in the freezer to set for at least 15 minutes.

5   To make the filling, put all the ingredients except the coconut oil in a food processor and blend together. With the motor still running, drizzle in the coconut oil. Pour the filling over the base, then tap the tin on the counter several times to ensure there are no air bubbles.

6   Scatter the chocolate shavings on top and return to the fridge for at least 3 hours to set.

7   This cake will keep in the fridge for up to a week and can be frozen for up to two months.

TIPS: If you've frozen the cake, defrost it in the fridge for at least 3 hours before serving.

You could easily make mini cakes in a mini loaf tin or muffin tin if you wanted to freeze smaller portions.

Sometimes you need something really special to wow people, and this cake does just that. If I'm invited to a friend's house for dinner I'll always offer to bring something, and a dessert is always well received. Bringing this cake to a party usually dismisses the view that vegan food is in any way bland or boring. This is rich, decadent and absolutely delicious.

Serves 10

FOR THE BASE:

melted coconut oil, for greasing

7 oz (200g) Medjool dates, pitted

3½ oz (100g) walnuts

approx. 1½ oz (40g) desiccated coconut

1 oz (30g) raw cacao power

FOR THE FILLING:

5¼ oz (150g) cashew nuts

2 ripe avocados, peeled and stoned

2 vanilla pods, cut in half lengthways and seeds scraped out, or ½ teaspoon vanilla powder

4 tablespoons raw cacao powder

4 tablespoons maple syrup

2 heaped tablespoons coconut sugar

2 tablespoons lucuma powder

2 tablespoons melted coconut oil

FOR THE TOPPING:

1 oz (30g) dark chocolate, shaved

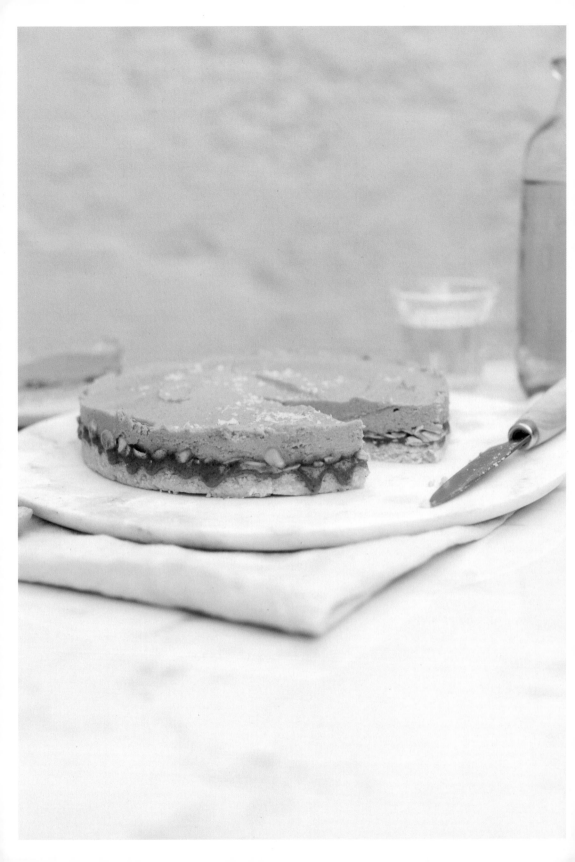

SALTED CARAMEL CELEBRATION CAKE

1   Put the 6⅓ oz (180g) of cashews for the top layer in a bowl, cover with filtered water and soak for at least 8 hours or ideally overnight. Drain and rinse, then pat them dry thoroughly with a clean tea towel or kitchen paper. (See the note on page 30 on soaking nuts.)

2   Preheat the oven to 285°F (140°C). Brush a thin layer of melted coconut oil over the base and sides of a 8" (20cm) tin.

3   Make the base by blitzing the nuts in a food processor until fine, but be careful not to over-blend or the nuts will start to release their oils. Add the desiccated coconut and coconut oil and pulse to combine, then add the sweetener and pulse again. Press this evenly onto the base of the greased cake tin, pushing it down firmly to make sure there are no gaps. I use the base of a glass to press it down.

4   Bake in the oven for 8 minutes. Set aside to cool on a wire rack.

5   To make the caramel layer, put the maple syrup and almond butter in a small saucepan set over a low heat and melt them together. Stir in the flaked almonds and salt. Spoon the caramel onto the middle of the base and spread it out, but keep ½ inch (1cm) clear around the edges. Put the base in the freezer for at least 15 minutes to set.

6   Make the top layer by combining all the ingredients except the salt in a food processor. Spoon on top of the caramel layer, then add a pinch of sea salt over the top. Return to the fridge to set for at least 3 hours before serving. Cut into slices with a sharp knife.

Of all the recipes in the book, this is the one that I'm most proud of. I love the sweetness of the caramel, the crunch of the nuts and the texture of the base.

Serves 10

FOR THE BASE:

approx. 4½ oz (125g) cashew nuts

4¼ oz (140g) desiccated coconut

1 teaspoon coconut oil, plus extra melted oil for greasing

¼ cup (50ml) maple or agave syrup

FOR THE CARAMEL LAYER:

3 tablespoons maple syrup

2 tablespoons almond butter

2⅖ oz (80g) flaked almonds

a pinch of Maldon flaky sea salt

FOR THE TOP LAYER:

6 oz (180g) cashew nuts

2 vanilla pods, cut in half lengthways and seeds scraped out, or ½ teaspoon vanilla extract

4 tablespoons coconut sugar

4 tablespoons coconut cream from a tin (see page 308)

3 tablespoons cacao butter or coconut oil, melted

2 tablespoons maple syrup

1 tablespoon maca powder

a pinch of Maldon flaky sea salt

PECAN BROWNIES WITH CASHEW ICING

A vegan brownie has connotations of something that's supposed to be nice, but isn't really. I've had my fair share of those kinds of brownie. But these are totally indulgent and delicious. I love the surprise of the nuts inside and the thick, creamy icing. If you want a real dessert, these will do the trick! I make them with oats which gives a really dense brownie, but if you want a lighter option feel free to substitute with brown rice or spelt flour.

Makes 12

7 oz (200g) oats or flour

9 oz (260g) dark soft brown sugar

7 oz (200g) raw cacao powder

1 teaspoon baking powder

1 teaspoon of vanilla essence

1 cup (250ml) of plant milk

1 ripe banana

1 tablespoon of chia seeds

6 oz (180g) coconut oil, melted, plus
   extra for greasing

2 oz (60g) pecans (or you could use
   flaked almonds or walnuts halves)

FOR THE CASHEW ICING:

4 tablespoons agave syrup

2 tablespoons cashew butter

1 vanilla pod, cut in half
   lengthways and seeds scraped out

1½ oz (40g) cacao butter, melted

1   Put the chia seeds and water in a bowl and stir to combine. Set them aside for about 10 minutes to allow the seeds to gel.

2   Preheat the oven to 350°F (170°C). Line a 9" x 9" (23cm x 23cm) baking tin with non-stick baking paper and lightly brush with a tiny bit of melted coconut oil.

3   If using oats, blitz the oats in a food processor for approximately 10 seconds until a fine flour is formed. Add the sugar, baking powder and cacao powder and blend to combine before adding in the wet ingredients and banana.

4   Pour the mixture into the lined tin. Shake the tin to ensure it fills all the spaces, then tap it on the counter a few times to ensure that there are no air bubbles. Scatter the pecans over the top, then shake the tin again and push them down into the batter.

5   Bake in the oven for 20 minutes. It will still be slightly soft in the middle. Allow to cool in the tin on a wire rack for 15 minutes while you make the icing.

6   To make the icing, blend the agave, cashew butter and vanilla together until well combined, then drizzle in the melted cacao butter and stir to combine.

7   Spread the icing over the cooled brownies, then put in the fridge to set. Cut into 12 squares and store in an airtight container in the fridge for up to five days.

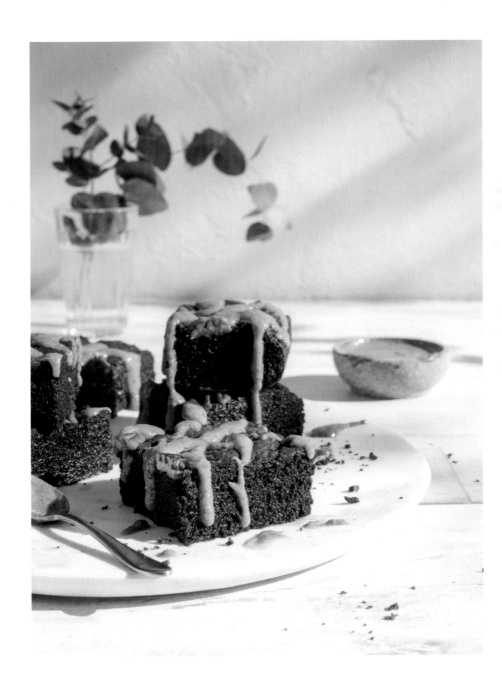

CARAMEL AND CHOCOLATE SLICES

I prefer these to almost any kind of chocolate bar you can buy, so I try to have some in my freezer all the time. Nothing is more satisfying than seeing friends dig into these, blissfully unaware that they are vegan, and then claim that they're the nicest caramel squares ever!

Makes 10

FOR THE BASE:

5 oz (140g) Medjool dates, pitted

3½ oz (100g) cashew nuts

3 oz (90g) desiccated coconut

1½ oz (40g) rolled oats

1 tablespoon melted coconut oil

FOR THE DATE CARAMEL:

7 oz (200g) Medjool dates, pitted

4 tablespoons almond or cashew butter

1 tablespoon melted coconut oil

a pinch of sea salt

FOR THE TOP LAYER:

3½ oz (100g) cacao butter

1½ oz (40g) raw cacao powder

¾ oz (20g) coconut sugar or 2 tablespoons agave syrup

a handful of flaked almonds (optional)

1   Put the dates, cashews, desiccated coconut and oats in a food processor and blend to combine.

2   Line a 7" x 8" (15cm x 20cm) baking tin with non-stick baking paper, then transfer the base mixture to the tin, pressing it down firmly with your hands or a spatula. Make sure you get it into all the corners. Put in the freezer to set.

3   Don't worry about cleaning the food processor in between – just scrape it out with a spatula. Put all the date caramel ingredients in the food processor and blend until smooth. Spread the caramel on top of the base and return to the freezer to set.

4   Create a double boiler by simmering a little water in a saucepan and placing a second pan or heatproof bowl on top, making sure the bottom of the pan or bowl doesn't touch the water. Put the cacao butter in the pan or bowl and allow to melt, then remove from the heat. Whisk in the cacao powder and coconut sugar until creamy. Pour the chocolate over the caramel layer. To add extra crunch, scatter some flaked almonds on top of the chocolate before you put it in the fridge to set.

5   Refrigerate for 3 hours before cutting into 10 slices. These will keep in an airtight container in the fridge for up to five days, but I also love these straight from the freezer, where they will keep for up to two months.

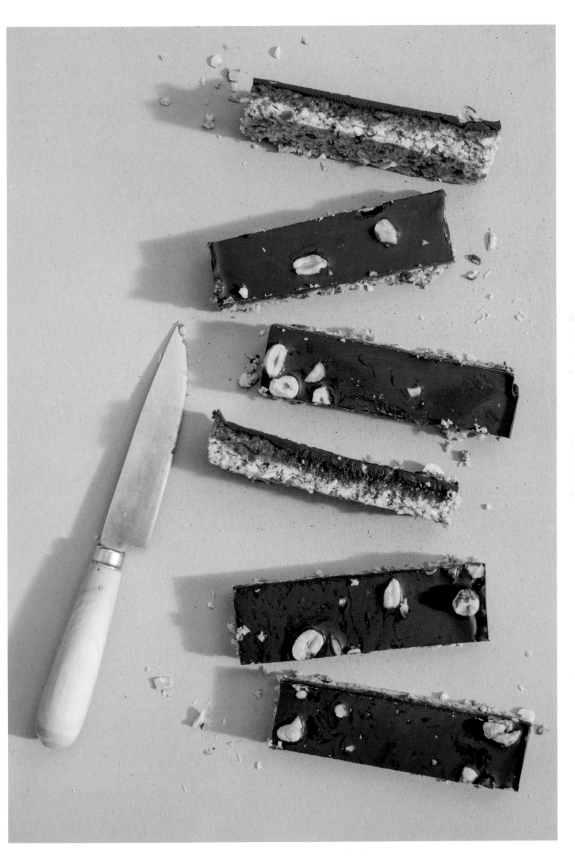

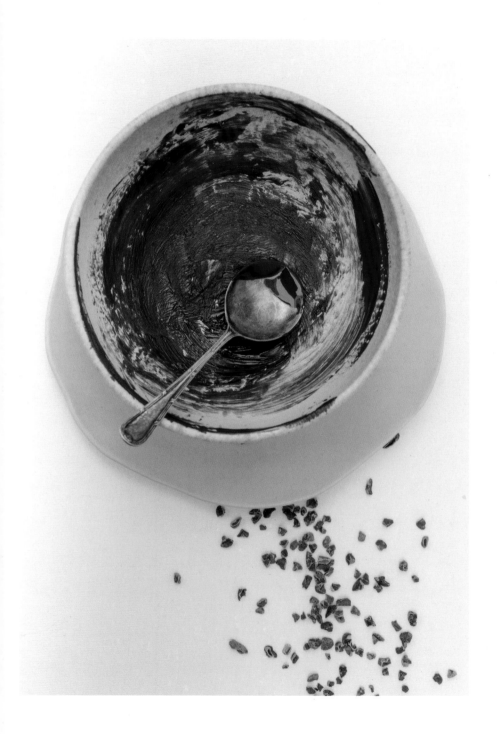

RAW CHOCOLATE MOUSSE WITH FLAKED ALMONDS

1 Put the cashews in a bowl, cover with filtered water and soak for at least 8 hours or ideally overnight. Drain and rinse, then pat them dry thoroughly with a clean tea towel or kitchen paper. (See the note on page 30 on soaking nuts.)

2 Lightly toast the almonds on a low heat in a dry pan. When they start to go lightly golden, remove them from the heat and tip them out onto a fresh plate to cool down. Put them in the fridge if you need them to cool faster.

3 Put all the ingredients except the almonds and shaved dark chocolate in a blender and blitz together until silky smooth. I like to serve these in ramekins, which is also a useful way to work out portions if you'll be freezing leftovers. Spoon the mousse into the ramekins and top with a pinch of the shaved chocolate and some of the flaked almonds. Feel free to add a tiny pinch of sea salt too.

4 Chill in the fridge for at least 3 hours before serving.

We all look forward to dessert, but telling people that you have made something healthy or mentioning that the mousse has avocado in it might dampen their enthusiasm. So say nothing and just enjoy the compliments that come your way once people taste this!

Serves 4

5 oz (150g) cashew nuts

2 ripe avocados, peeled and stoned

2 vanilla pods, cut in half lengthways and seeds scraped out, or ½ teaspoon vanilla powder

4 tablespoons raw cacao powder

3 tablespoons maple syrup

2 heaped tablespoons coconut sugar

2 tablespoons lucuma powder

2 tablespoons coconut oil

FOR THE TOPPING:

1 oz (30g) flaked almonds

1 oz (30g) dark chocolate, shaved

a pinch of sea salt (optional)

CARAMEL CASHEW MOUSSE WITH RAW CHOCOLATE LACE

The combination of maple syrup, coconut sugar and maca powder gives this dessert a rich caramel flavour – when I first made it, I was blown away by the taste. Adding the chocolate lace makes it an even more special dessert.

Serves 4

6 oz (180g) cashew nuts

2 vanilla pods, cut in half lengthways and seeds scraped out, or ½ teaspoon vanilla extract

4 tablespoons coconut cream from a tin (see page 308)

3 tablespoons cacao butter or coconut oil, melted

4 tablespoons coconut sugar

2 tablespoons maple syrup

1 tablespoon maca powder

FOR THE RAW CHOCOLATE LACE:

2 tablespoons maple syrup

1 tablespoon cacao butter, melted

2 tablespoons raw cacao powder

¾ oz (20g) cacao nibs

1   Put the cashews in a bowl, cover with filtered water and soak for at least 8 hours or ideally overnight. Drain and rinse, then pat them dry thoroughly with a clean tea towel or kitchen paper. (See the note on page 30 on soaking nuts.)

2   To make the chocolate lace, line a large plate or baking tray – whatever size will fit in your freezer – with non-stick baking paper.

3   Create a double boiler by simmering a little water in a saucepan and placing a second pan or heatproof bowl on top, making sure the bottom of the pan or bowl doesn't touch the water. Put the maple syrup and cacao butter in the pan or bowl and allow them to melt together. Remove from the heat, then quickly whisk in the cacao powder. Once combined, drizzle the chocolate on the baking paper in lacy patterns. Top with the cacao nibs and put in the freezer to set.

4   To make the mousse, put all the ingredients in a blender and combine until silky smooth. Pour the mousse into the bowl you will be serving it in or individual ramekins or mini bowls. Put in the fridge for at least 2 hours to set.

5   When ready to serve, decorate with pieces of the chocolate lace. The mousse will keep in the fridge for up to three days and the chocolate lace will keep in the freezer for up to two months.

VANILLA CASHEW MOUSSE WITH BLUEBERRY COULIS

1   Put the cashews in a bowl, cover with filtered water and soak for at least 8 hours or ideally overnight. Drain and rinse, then pat them dry thoroughly with a clean tea towel or kitchen paper. (See the note on page 30 on soaking nuts.)

2   To make the mousse, put all the ingredients except the coconut water in a blender and combine until silky smooth. Add a splash of coconut water if it's not coming together. Pour the mousse into the bowl you will be serving it in or individual ramekins or mini bowls. Put in the fridge for at least 2 hours to set.

3   To make the blueberry coulis, blend the blueberries, agave syrup, chia seeds and lemon juice together until smooth. With the motor still running, drizzle in the melted coconut oil.

4   Once the mousse has set, drizzle the coulis over the top and return to the fridge for at least another 3 hours to set.

5   Serve with fresh blueberries scattered on top. The mousse will keep in the fridge for up to four days.

TIP: Use light agave syrup, not dark, or the colour will be light brown, which isn't as pretty.

This vanilla mousse is the perfect partner for any in-season fruit. I love the contrast of the blueberries but you can use any berries, stewed fruit or even chocolate or cacao nibs to dress it up.

Serves 4

6 oz (180g) cashew nuts

1¾ oz (50g) desiccated coconut

2 vanilla pods, cut in half lengthways and seeds scraped out, or ½ teaspoon vanilla extract

3 tablespoons coconut cream from a tin (see page 308)

3 tablespoons light agave syrup

3 tablespoons cacao butter or coconut oil, melted

2 tablespoons maple syrup

1 tablespoon maca powder

splash of coconut water, if needed

FOR THE BLUEBERRY COULIS:

3½ oz (100g) fresh or frozen blueberries, plus extra fresh berries to serve

2 tablespoons agave syrup

1 teaspoon chia seeds

1 teaspoon lemon juice

1 teaspoon melted coconut oil

RASPBERRY AND CUSTARD TART

You need fresh raspberries for these tarts. You can use any type of berry that you like or whatever is in season, but frozen berries release too much liquid, which would make the base soggy and likely to fall apart.

Serves 4

5 oz (150g) fresh raspberries, washed and dried as thoroughly as possible

FOR THE TART CASE:

1 teaspoon melted coconut oil

4½ oz (125g) cashew nuts

5 oz (120g) desiccated coconut

4 tablespoons maple or agave syrup

a pinch of sea salt

FOR THE CUSTARD:

3 oz (80g) cashew nuts

1 vanilla pod, cut in half lengthways and seeds scraped out

2 tablespoons coconut cream from a tin (see page 308)

2 tablespoons maple or agave syrup

1 teaspoon coconut oil

1   Put the 3 oz (80g) of cashews for the filling in a bowl, cover with filtered water and soak for at least 8 hours or ideally overnight. Drain and rinse, then pat them dry thoroughly with a clean tea towel or kitchen paper. (See the note on page 30 on soaking nuts.)

2   Brush a thin layer of the melted coconut oil over the base and sides of a 6" (15cm) springform tin.

3   To make the base, start by blending the approx. 4½ oz (125g) of cashews in a food processor until fine, but be careful not to over-blend or else the nuts will start to release their oils. Add the desiccated coconut and pulse to combine, then drizzle in the sweetener and blend again. Press this evenly onto the base and up the sides of the greased tin, pushing it down firmly to make sure there are no gaps. I use the base of a glass to press it down and ensure the edges are firm. Put it in the freezer to set for at least 30 minutes.

4   To make the custard, combine all the ingredients in a blender until smooth. Spoon the custard on top of the base and put in the fridge to set for at least 30 minutes before topping with the fresh raspberries. Once assembled, store in the fridge but ideally serve as soon as possible to ensure the base stays firm.

LIME TART WITH RASPBERRY COMPOTE

1   Put the cashews in a bowl, cover with filtered water and soak for at least 8 hours or ideally overnight. Drain and rinse, then pat them dry thoroughly with a clean tea towel or kitchen paper. (See the note on page 30 on soaking nuts.)

2   Line a 6" (15cm) springform baking tin with non-stick baking paper and lightly grease with coconut oil.

3   To make the base, blend the nut flour and desiccated coconut together in a food processor, then drizzle in the agave syrup. Press this evenly onto the base of the prepared tin and about ½ inch (1cm) up the sides, pushing it down firmly to make sure there are no gaps. Use the base of a glass or the heel of your hand to press it down.

4   You can freeze this for about 20 minutes, until set, if you want to keep it raw, but I like to bake it for about 10 minutes at 285°F (140°C), which makes it a little crisp and golden.

5   To make the filling, zest both of the limes and juice one lime. Cut off any remaining pith or peel from the remaining lime after you've zested it, then cut that lime into slices. Put the lime zest, juice and slices in the food processor with the rest of the filling ingredients and blend together until silky smooth. Taste it to see if you're happy with the sharpness, adding a little more lime juice or sweetener depending on your preference. Pour the filling into the tart case and refrigerate for 3 hours to set.

(continued)

This is the kind of dessert that leaves you feeling so satisfied, but the refreshing lime zest is fresh and light. **Makes 1 x 20cm cake**

FOR THE BASE:

coconut oil, for greasing

4½ oz (125g) nut flour – grind any nuts to a flour-like consistency (I use almonds)

5 oz (120g) desiccated coconut

4 tablespoons agave syrup

FOR THE LIME FILLING:

2 limes

3 oz (80g) coconut butter or 1 ripe avocado

approx. 1½ oz (40g) cashew nuts

4 tablespoons agave syrup

2 tablespoons coconut oil

FOR THE RASPBERRY COMPOTE:

5 oz (120g) frozen raspberries

4¼ fl oz (125ml) filtered water

1 tablespoon chia seeds

1 tablespoon lemon juice

1 tablespoon agave syrup

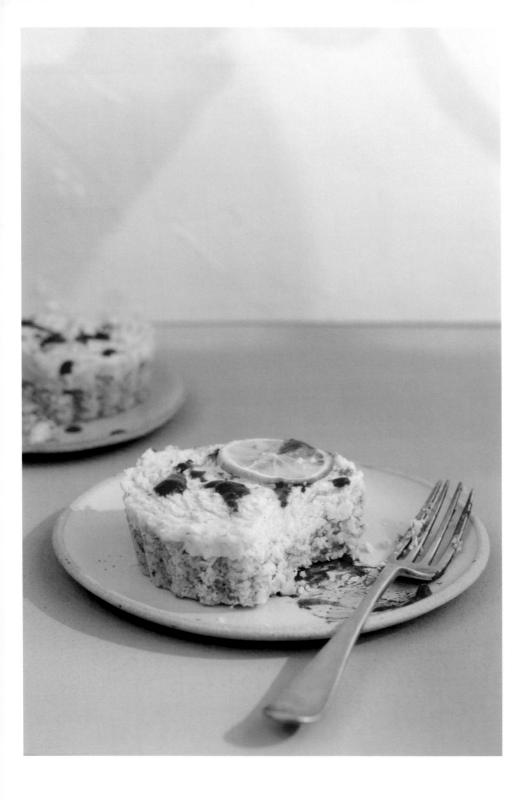

6 To make the raspberry compote, put the berries and water in a small saucepan and simmer for 10 minutes. When the berries are starting to soften, add the chia seeds, lemon juice and agave syrup. Remove from the heat and allow to cool for 10 minutes. Use a hand-held blender or pour it into a blender and process it to a creamy consistency.

7 Serve each slice of the lime tart with a generous helping of the raspberry compote on the side.

TIP: Coconut butter is thick, sweet, and very creamy. It includes the meat of the coconut, while coconut oil does not. The cocount meat is slowly dried to help ensure as much of the delicious tropical flavour is retained. Coconut butter should be available in all heath food stores.

PASSION FRUIT AND LIME PIE

I've always loved the freshness of citrus as a dessert. It feels like a light way to end a meal while still ticking the box for sweetness. I like this tart to be quite sharp so that when it's served with the coconut cream it creates a nice sweet and sour contrast, but feel free to add another 1–2 tablespoons of agave syrup to the filling if you'd like it to be sweeter – if you'll be serving this to children, I would definitely do this.

Serves 10

FOR THE BASE:

melted coconut oil, for greasing

5 oz (150g) cashew nuts

5 oz (150g) macadamia nuts

3 oz (80g) desiccated coconut

2⅔ oz (75g) Medjool dates, pitted

2 fl oz (60ml) maple syrup

FOR THE FILLING:

2 limes

7 oz (200g) cashew nuts

5 oz (150g) coconut oil, melted

1 ripe avocado, peeled and stoned

juice of 1 lemon

4 tablespoons maple or agave syrup, plus extra to taste and for drizzling

1 tablespoon maca powder

1 teaspoon vanilla extract

3 passion fruits

TO SERVE:

vanilla coconut cream (page 309)

1 Put the 7 oz (200g) of cashews for the filling in a bowl, cover with filtered water and soak for at least 8 hours or ideally overnight. Drain and rinse, then pat them dry thoroughly with a clean tea towel or kitchen paper. (See the note on page 30 on soaking nuts.)

2 Brush a thin layer of melted coconut oil over the base and sides of a 8" (20cm) loose-bottomed cake tin.

3 Put all the base ingredients in a food processor and blend to combine. Press this evenly onto the base of the greased cake tin, pushing it down firmly to make sure there are no gaps. I use the base of a glass to press it down. Put it in the freezer to set for at least 15 minutes.

4 To make the filling, zest both of the limes. Cut off any remaining pith or peel after you've zested them, then cut the limes into slices. Set aside 1 teaspoon of the lime zest, then put the remaining zest, the lime slices and all the other filling ingredients except the passion fruit in a food processor and blend until well combined. Taste it and if you want to add more sweetness, drizzle in more maple or agave syrup a tablespoon at a time. When you're happy with the sweetness, scoop out the passion fruit flesh and pulse briefly or fold it in to combine.

5 Pour the filling onto the base layer, then tap the tin against the counter a few times to ensure there are no air bubbles. Put in the fridge for at least 2 hours to set.

6 To serve, add a drizzle of agave syrup and sprinkle over the reserved lime zest. Cut into slices and serve with a dollop of vanilla coconut cream.

7 This will keep in the fridge for up to 10 days or in the freezer for up to two months.

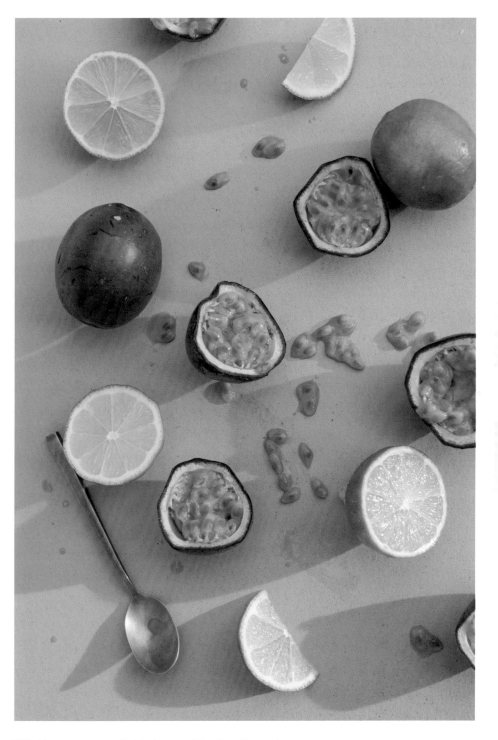

TIP: Always zest citrus fruit before you juice it, as it's much easier to do while they're still whole and firm.

ETON MESS

I first tasted a vegan Eton mess when I travelled to Thailand. Through the power of social media I found some incredible restaurants and one had an Eton mess sundae. Falling in love with a dessert that you had on the other side of the world is always a great motivation to try to recreate it at home! Set against a backdrop of fresh berries, vanilla coconut cream and some flaked almonds for texture, this is as good as a summer dessert gets.

Serves 2

coconut oil, for greasing

FOR THE VEGAN MERINGUES:
1 x 14 oz (400g) tin of chickpeas, drained and aquafaba reserved
3½ oz (100g) caster sugar

FOR THE VANILLA CASHEW CREAM:
4½ oz (125g) cashews
2 tablespoons maple or agave syrup
1 vanilla pod, cut in half lengthways and seeds scraped out
6¾ fl oz (200ml) filtered water

TO SERVE:
3½ oz (100g) fresh berries or fruit per person
3 oz (80g) toasted flaked almonds

1   Put the cashews in a bowl, cover with filtered water and soak for at least 8 hours or ideally overnight. Drain and rinse, then pat them dry thoroughly with a clean tea towel or kitchen paper. (See the note on page 30 on soaking nuts.)

2   Preheat the oven to 350°F (180°C). Line a baking tray with non-stick baking paper, then lightly grease it with a little coconut oil.

3   Make your meringues by putting the aquafaba in a medium-sized mixing bowl and whisking to soft peaks, just like egg whites. Add the sugar very slowly, whisking constantly, until thick and glossy. Spoon or pipe the meringue onto the lined tray in blobs about 1" (2.5cm) wide. Bake in the oven for 1 hour 15 minutes, until crisp. Allow to cool completely before breaking the meringues into bite-sized pieces.

4   Make the cashew cream by putting the soaked cashews in a high-powered blender and blitzing to a thick paste. Add the maple or agave syrup and the vanilla seeds and blend to combine before slowly drizzling in the water with the motor running until your desired consistency is reached. I like this to be thick. Store in the fridge in an airtight container until you're ready to serve.

5   To serve, layer the broken meringues on a plate and pile the fruit, vanilla cashew cream and toasted flaked almonds on top.

TIP: I serve this on plates, but if you have sundae glasses this will look amazing in them!

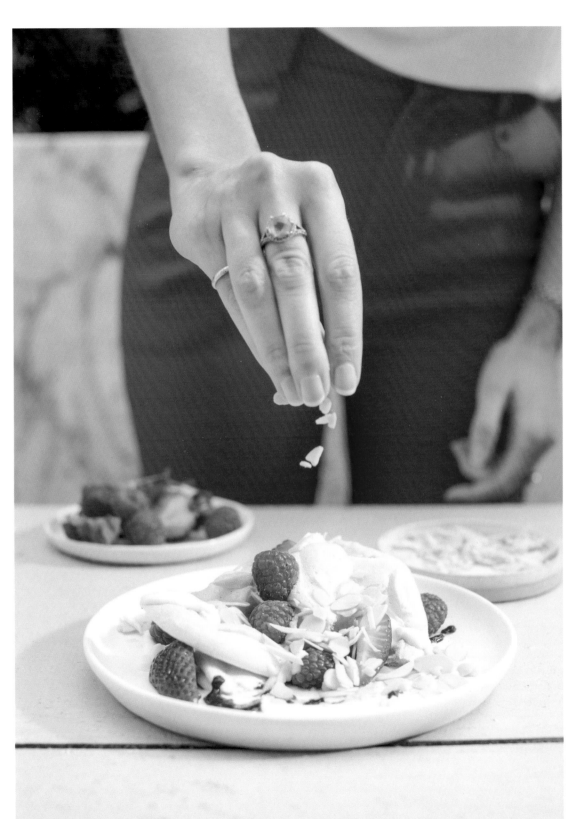

BERRIES WITH WARM VANILLA SAUCE

You can make this with fresh or frozen berries, whatever suits. If you're using fresh berries, keep them well chilled, as what's lovely about this dish is the contrast of warm and cool. If you're using frozen berries, take them out of the freezer and allow to thaw for about 15 minutes, otherwise they will be too hard to eat.

Serves 2

7 oz (200g) chilled or frozen berries
3½ oz (100g) flaked almonds

FOR THE WARM VANILLA SAUCE:

3 tablespoons cashew butter
6 tablespoons coconut sugar
3 tablespoons almond milk
1 vanilla pod, cut in half lengthways
   and seeds scraped out
a pinch of sea salt
1½ oz (40g) cacao butter, melted

1   Put all the sauce ingredients except the melted cacao butter in a blender and blitz to combine. With the motor still running, drizzle in the melted cacao butter until well combined, but don't over-blend or it will separate.

2   Create a double boiler by simmering a little water in a saucepan and placing a second pan or heatproof bowl on top, making sure the bottom of the pan or bowl doesn't touch the water. Put the sauce in the pan or bowl to warm it gently prior to serving.

3   Remove the chilled berries from the fridge or allow frozen berries to thaw for 15 minutes before serving. Transfer the frozen berries to two room temperature serving bowls, as bowls that are too cold could crack from the heat of the warm sauce.

4   Drizzle the sauce over the berries and top with the flaked almonds.

TIP: You can make the vanilla sauce in advance – just keep it warm over a double boiler on a low heat.

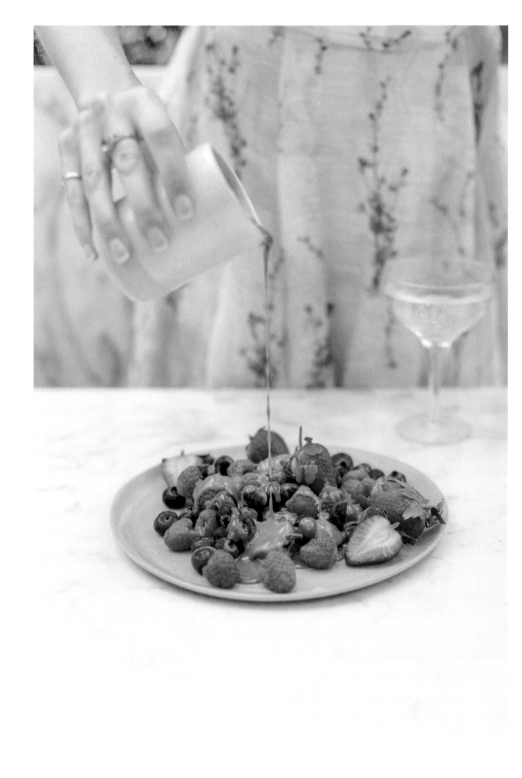

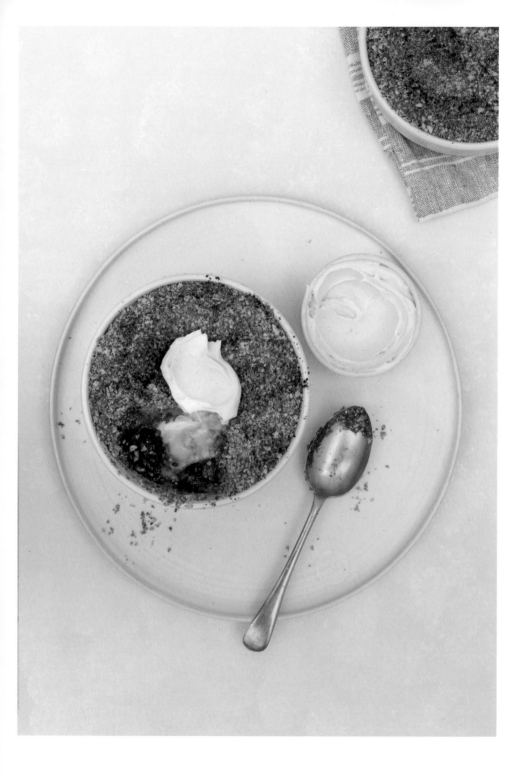

MIXED BERRY AND APPLE CRUMBLE WITH VANILLA COCONUT CREAM

1   Preheat the oven to 325°F (160°C).

2   Put the apples, berries, coconut sugar, apple or orange juice, lemon juice, cornflour and cinnamon in a large bowl and mix together, making sure the apples and berries are all coated with the juice and cornflour. Drizzle in a little maple syrup if you think the fruit is too tart.

3   Transfer to a baking dish.

4   Put all the crumble ingredients in a medium-sized bowl and mix together, then pat it on top of the apple and berry mix.

5   Bake in the oven for 50 minutes. Finish it under the grill for the last few minutes to crisp it up. It will be piping hot, so I let it stand for 10 minutes before serving.

6   When the coconut cream hits the heat of the crumble it will melt straight away, so keep it chilled in the fridge and allow people to help themselves to keep it cool until the last minute.

It's easy to vary the fruit in a crumble depending on what you have or what's in season or on special offer in your supermarket. I love the simplicity of berries and apples, but you could also try peaches or rhubarb.

Serves 4

4 apples, peeled, cored and chopped

7 oz (200g) fresh or frozen mixed
   berries

3½ oz (100g) coconut sugar

approx. 3⅓ fl oz (100ml) apple or
   orange juice

juice of 1 lemon

1 tablespoon cornflour

1 heaped teaspoon ground cinnamon

maple syrup to sweeten (optional)

FOR THE CRUMBLE TOPPING:

3½ oz (100g) rolled oats

3½ oz (100g) coconut sugar

2 oz (50g) ground almonds

2 oz (50g) flaked almonds

5 tablespoons melted coconut oil

TO SERVE:

vanilla coconut cream (page 309)

CHARGRILLED PINEAPPLE WITH CARAMEL SAUCE

This is a perfect summer dessert with a surprisingly easy-to-make caramel sauce. This one is rich, sweet and creamy. It naturally thickens after being left in the fridge if you're making it in advance, so if you want to thin it down, use a little plant-based milk to bring it back to the consistency you like. This is a versatile sauce, so try it over other fruit or spooned over ice cream.

Serves 4

1 ripe pineapple

coconut oil, for grilling

coconut or caster sugar, for dusting

1 batch of caramel sauce (page 310), to serve

1   To grill the pineapple, cut off the top and bottom and discard. Cut the pineapple in half lengthways, then quarter it, then cut again into long wedges. Remove the woody core in the middle. This is often much whiter and firmer than the flesh, so it should be easy to see where to cut. Cut away the skin as close to the flesh as possible.

2   Heat a little coconut oil in a chargrill pan set over a high heat. Put the pineapple wedges in the hot pan and allow to cook for 2 minutes before turning to allow nice grill marks to form. Dust the grilled sides with a little coconut sugar and continue to cook for 3–4 minutes more, until the other sides have grill marks too and have heated through.

3   Transfer to a warmed plate and drizzle with the caramel sauce before serving.

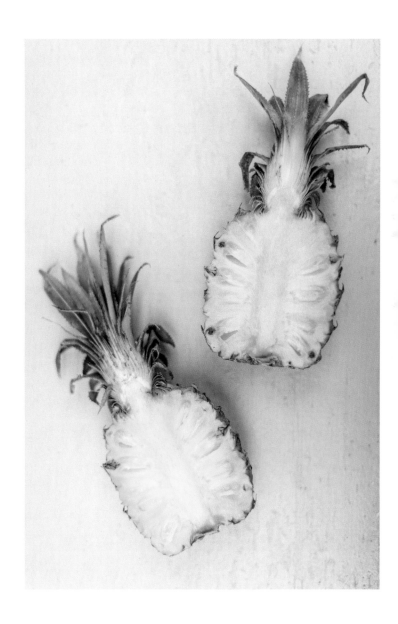

RAW CHOCOLATE AND FREEZE-DRIED RASPBERRY SHERBET TRUFFLES

Basic raw chocolate is the perfect way to inject flavour and use up any odds and ends of dried fruit you might have in your cupboards. They elevate something simple to something really special.

You'll need a silicone chocolate mould for this.

Makes approx. 25 truffles

2 heaped teaspoons freeze-dried raspberry powder, plus extra for dusting

3½ oz (100g) cacao butter

approx. 1½ oz (40g) raw cacao powder

¾ oz (20g) coconut sugar

1 Add a small dusting of raspberry powder to each of the moulds.

2 Create a double boiler by simmering a little water in a saucepan and placing a second pan or heatproof bowl on top, making sure the bottom of the pan or bowl doesn't touch the water.

3 Put the cacao butter in the pan or bowl and allow to melt, then remove from the heat. Whisk in the cacao powder and coconut sugar together until creamy. Add the raspberry powder and whisk again to combine.

4 Pour into the chocolate moulds. Sift a light dusting of raspberry powder over them before placing in the freezer to set for at least 1 hour. Store the truffles in the freezer for up to two months.

TIP: Freeze-dried raspberry powder can be hard to find, but it's phenomenal and a little goes a long way.

CRUNCHY MACA FUDGE

1 Blend the dates and macadamia nuts until smooth. Transfer to a mixing bowl, then add the quinoa pops an maca powder and knead the mixture with your hands.

2 Line an airtight container or small baking tray (the one I use is 6" [15cm] long) with non-stick baking paper. Spread the fudge mixture out and flatten it into an even layer. Freeze for at least 4 hours.

3 Cut into small squares, as it is quite a sweet treat and a little goes a long way. Keep in the freezer in an airtight container for up to two months.

This is lovely crumbled over plain vanilla yogurt or anything you want to add a little more sweetness to.

Makes about 18 squares

6½ oz (185g) Medjool dates, pitted

5 oz (140g) macadamia nuts

1 oz (30g) quinoa pops

1 tablespoon maca powder

It's always reassuring to have a few snacks
to hand. Whether you want energy balls to take
with you, something sweet like cookies or the
most delicious kale crisps you will ever have,
it's all in here.

SNACKS

CRISPY KALE CRUNCHIES

You haven't tried kale crisps until you've tried these! I make as many as my dehydrator tray will allow at a time. I'm slightly ashamed to admit that I hide them, as these are one thing I don't like sharing.

They can be enjoyed on their own or else they make a lovely crunchy topping to simple dishes like the mac and cheese on page 145 or salads.

Serves 4

3½ oz (100g) cashew nuts

3 fl oz (100ml) filtered water

7 oz (200g) kale

3 tablespoons nutritional yeast

2 tablespoons raw apple cider vinegar or lemon juice

2 tablespoons olive oil, plus extra for greasing

3½ oz (100g) of finely chopped shallots

1 teaspoon of onion powder

1 teaspoon ground turmeric

¼ teaspoon cayenne pepper

sea salt and freshly ground black pepper

1 Put the cashews in a bowl, cover with filtered water and soak for at least 8 hours or ideally overnight. Drain and rinse, then pat them dry thoroughly with a clean tea towel or kitchen paper. (See the note on page 30 on soaking nuts.)

2 Preheat the oven to 300°F (150°C). Line a large baking tray with non-stick baking paper and lightly oil it. Alternatively, you can use a dehydrator for this if you have one.

3 Strip the kale leaves from the thick rib and wash the leaves. Dry them in a salad spinner or pat them dry as thoroughly as possible so that the sauce will stick to them later on.

4 Put the soaked cashews, nutritional yeast, vinegar or lemon juice, olive oil, shallots and all the herbs with a pinch of salt and pepper in a high-powered blender and blend until silky smooth, drizzling in the water as required.

5 Put the kale leaves in a large bowl, then pour in the sauce. Use your hands to massage the sauce into the kale really well, making sure each piece of kale is covered.

6 Spread the kale out on the baking tray and bake in the oven for 20–30 minutes. Halfway through the cooking time, rotate the tray and move some of the kale in the centre towards the edge so that it cooks evenly. After this you should check on it every 5 minutes, as the kale can burn very quickly.

7 If you're using a dehydrator, spread the kale out on one or two trays and cook for 6 hours or even overnight at 175°F (80°C). If you want to keep them raw, set the temperature to 110°F (42°C) and leave them to dehydrate for 24 hours, until crisp.

8 Allow the kale crisps to stand for 10 minutes once they're out of the oven before digging in. This helps the flavours set into them. Store in an airtight container for up to five days.

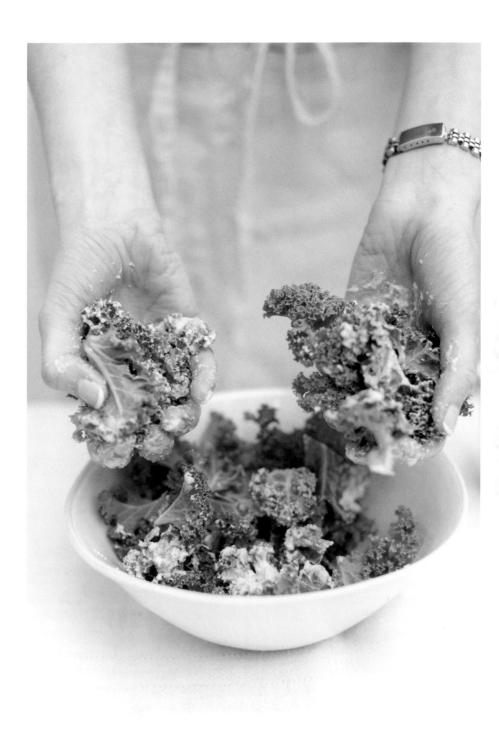

SWEET POTATO CRISPS

Making your own crisps is one of those rainy day things to do. They don't need a lot of prep, but you do need to monitor them and the only real hassle is turning each crisp over individually. I make these in large batches, as knowing I have a large stash to enjoy makes the effort worthwhile.

Serves 6

6 large sweet potatoes

1 tablespoon olive oil, plus extra for greasing

1 teaspoon tamari, soy sauce or coconut aminos

fine sea salt and freshly ground black pepper

1   Preheat the oven to 285°F (140°C). Line two baking trays with tin foil and lightly grease them with a little olive oil.

2   Thoroughly wash and scrub your potatoes (I don't bother peeling them). Ensure they are completely dry. Using a mandoline, a peeler or the thinnest setting on your food processor, slice them very thinly.

3   Put the olive oil and tamari in a mixing bowl and whisk together. Add the potato slices and make sure they are all evenly coated on both sides.

4   Put the crisps on the greased trays. Make sure they aren't clumped together, as this will make them go soggy. Bake in the oven for 1 hour, then remove the trays from the oven, turn each crisp over and bake for a further 20 minutes or so. If they aren't as golden brown as you would like at this stage, put them under the grill for approximately 3 minutes.

5   Sprinkle with salt and pepper and allow to cool before enjoying.

6   These will last for up to a week in an airtight container. If they go a little soft, return them to a hot oven for 4–6 minutes to crisp them up again.

TIP: These go really well with guacamole (page 241) or one of my hummus recipes (pages 244–246).

MACA AND CRANBERRY ENERGY BALLS

1 Put the cashews and maca powder in a food processor. Blitz for about 20 seconds, until the nuts are all broken down. Add the dates a few at a time and blend well. Add the coconut oil and blend again, then add the cranberries and blend for about 10 seconds.

2 Take small handfuls of the mixture and roll it between your hands to form 10 small balls. Refrigerate for 20 minutes to allow the coconut oil to set.

3 Store in an airtight container in the fridge for up to 10 days or in the freezer for up to two months.

Energy balls are a really useful thing to have on hand. They can be expensive to buy but are surprisingly easy to make and customise. The addition of maca here will require a trip to a health food store, but it has a gorgeous sweet flavour.

Makes 10

7 oz (200g) cashew nuts

1 tablespoon maca powder

6 oz (180g) Medjool dates, pitted

1¾ oz (50g) dried cranberries

1 teaspoon coconut oil, at room
    temperature

DATE AND NUT COOKIES

If you're looking for a grain-free cookie, I have the solution. These are so satisfying and really fill you up. You can customise the flavours here – try adding dried fruit instead of chocolate.

Makes 10

1 tablespoon chia seeds

1 tablespoon filtered water

3½ oz (100g) pecans

3 oz (85g) almonds

2 oz (60g) cacao nibs

3½ oz (100g) Medjool dates, pitted

2¾ fl oz (80ml) melted coconut oil, plus extra for greasing

1 vanilla pod, cut in half lengthways and seeds scraped out

1 tablespoon maca powder

1   Preheat the oven to 325°F (160°C). Grease a baking sheet with a little coconut oil.

2   Put the chia seeds and water in a small bowl and set aside for 10 minutes to gel.

3   Blend the pecans, almonds and cacao nibs together until a fine flour is formed. Add the dates, melted coconut oil, vanilla seeds, maca powder and the chia 'egg'. Process until everything has bound together into a dough. Break off portions about the size of a ping pong ball, then mould and flatten into a cookie shape.

4   Put the cookies on the greased baking sheet and bake in the oven for 20–30 minutes. I like them to be a little soft in the middle so I bake mine for only 20 minutes, but bake them for up to 30 minutes if you want a harder cookie. Allow to cool on a wire rack.

5   Store the cookies in an airtight container in the fridge for up to five days. I like to heat them up in a warm oven for a few minutes when I want to eat them. They are also delicious dipped into almond butter.

CACAO, COCONUT AND CHIA COOKIES

1 Put the chia seeds and water in a bowl and stir to combine. Set aside for about 10 minutes to allow the seeds to gel.

2 Preheat the oven to 350°F (180°C). Line a baking tray with non-stick baking paper and lightly grease with coconut oil.

3 Put the oats in a food processor and blend until a fine flour is formed. Add the hazelnuts, dates, cacao powder, syrup and desiccated coconut and blend to combine. Add the coconut oil and chia 'egg' and blend again. A ball of dough should form.

4 Using an ice cream scoop or spoon, take out a piece of dough about half the size of a golf ball and pat it between your palms until you get an even, flat biscuit shape. This will be messy, which is why it helps to have the oven on and the tray lined and ready! Place on the tray as you go.

5 Bake in the oven for 25 minutes. Allow to cool on a wire rack.

6 Store the cookies in an airtight container for up to five days. I like to keep them in the fridge, as it makes them a bit fudgy. If they go a little soft, put them on a baking tray in a warm oven for a few minutes.

Sometimes all you need is a really good cookie. Whether it's to be crumbled over some dairy-free ice cream or enjoyed with a cup of tea, if you're craving something really chocolatey, these will hit the spot!

When making these you can't help but notice that they are nutrient dense as well as delicious. You will be surprised how filling they are. I love them with a little bit of vanilla cashew butter spread on top.

Makes 10 large cookies

2 tablespoons chia seeds

6 tablespoons filtered water

7 oz (200g) jumbo oats

6 oz (180g) hazelnuts

5 Medjool dates, pitted

3 heaped tablespoons raw cacao powder

2 tablespoons agave or date syrup

1 tablespoon desiccated coconut

2 tablespoons coconut oil, plus extra for greasing

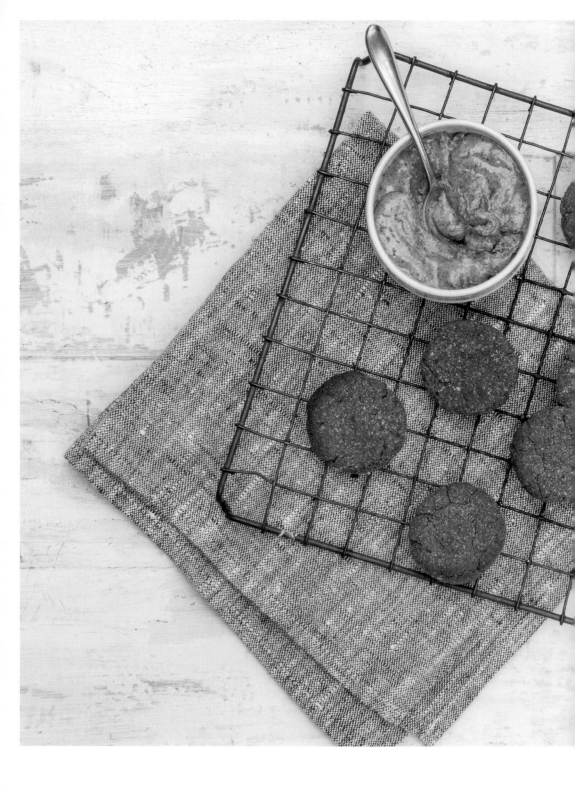

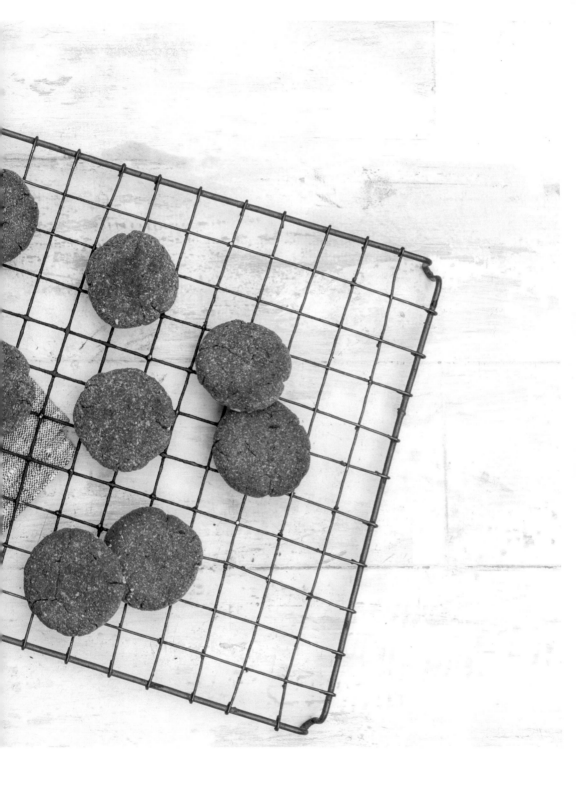

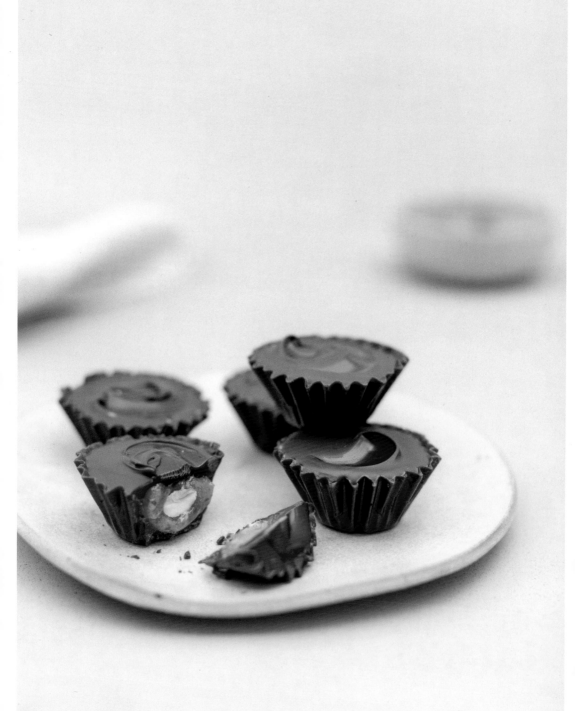

SALTED CARAMEL CHOCOLATE CUPS

1   A silicone mini muffin tin works best for these, but if you don't have one, line a 12-hole mini muffin tin with paper cases.

2   Create a double boiler by simmering a little water in a saucepan and placing a second pan or heatproof bowl on top, making sure the bottom of the pan or bowl doesn't touch the water. Break the chocolate into pieces and melt it in the bowl.

3   Pour a spoonful of melted chocolate into the bottom of each hole in the muffin tin. Bring it up on the sides of the mould with the back of a spoon or a pastry brush. Put the tin in the freezer for at least 20 minutes to allow the chocolate to set. Keep the rest of the melted chocolate warm and melted, as you will be using it again soon.

4   Meanwhile, make the caramel by melting the coconut oil in a small saucepan set over a medium heat. Add the almond butter and maple or agave syrup and stir continuously for about 2 minutes to combine. Don't be tempted to taste this while it's in the pan, as it gets really hot! Remove from the heat and stir in the coconut cream, oats and a small pinch of salt and stir to blend it all together. It should be a thick paste. Leave it to set and thicken for about 5 minutes.

5   Remove the muffin tin from the freezer. Working quickly, spoon ½ teaspoon of the caramel on top of all the chocolate cups. Press one almond into the caramel in each cup. Top with the remaining melted chocolate and return to the fridge for at least 1 hour to set.

6   Store in an airtight container in the fridge for up to 10 days or the freezer for up to two months.

There are very few vegan chocolates you can buy easily and they are often quite expensive. These are a real treat and are very easy to make. I had to hide them in the freezer, as the temptation to reach for another, and then another, became too much!

Makes 12

7 oz (200g) good-quality vegan dark chocolate, minimum 70% cocoa solids

1 teaspoon coconut oil

2 tablespoons almond butter

1 tablespoon maple or agave syrup

1 tablespoon vanilla coconut cream (see page 309)

1 heaped teaspoon oats

a pinch of sea salt

12 almonds

Whether you're adding some beetroot hummus to a piping hot baked potato, some miso dressing to a simple stir-fry or a dollop of vegan pesto to a plate of pasta, these are simple, easy additions that elevate the flavours of whatever you are making.

DIPS & DRESSINGS

TAHINI DRESSING

Tahini is a sesame seed paste that has a really thick, creamy texture and a taste that contrasts sharply with the cider vinegar or lemon in this dressing. It works particularly well served over roasted root vegetables or sweet potatoes.

Makes 6¾ fl oz (200ml)

1 teaspoon raw apple cider vinegar
   or lemon juice
1 tablespoon tahini
1 tablespoon nutritional yeast
1 tablespoon olive oil
1 teaspoon tamari, soy sauce or
   coconut aminos
6¾ fl oz (200ml) just-boiled water

1   Pour the apple cider vinegar or lemon juice over the tahini in a medium-sized bowl and use the back of a spoon or fork to break it down to a thinner consistency. When all the lumps are gone, add the nutritional yeast, olive oil and tamari. Add the hot water a little at a time to thin it to your desired consistency.

2   Store in a tightly sealed jar in the fridge for up to two weeks.

MISO DRESSING

1 Whisk the just-boiled water and almond butter together until it's a thin paste. Stir in the miso and blend again, then whisk in the olive oil and lemon juice. Season to taste with salt and pepper.
2 Store in a tightly sealed jar in the fridge for up to two weeks.

This effortless dressing injects flavour into simple veggies and elevates them on the taste scale phenomenally quickly. I like to pour this over a quick stir-fry or warm salad.

Makes 6¾ fl oz (200ml)

3⅓ fl oz (100ml) just-boiled water
1 tablespoon almond butter
1 large teaspoon miso paste
1 tablespoon olive oil
a squeeze of lemon juice
sea salt and freshly ground
  black pepper

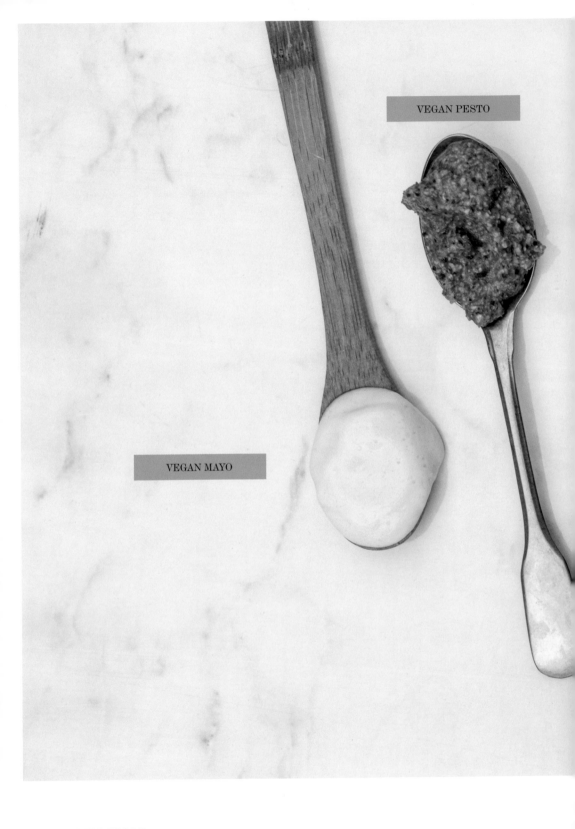

VEGAN PESTO

VEGAN MAYO

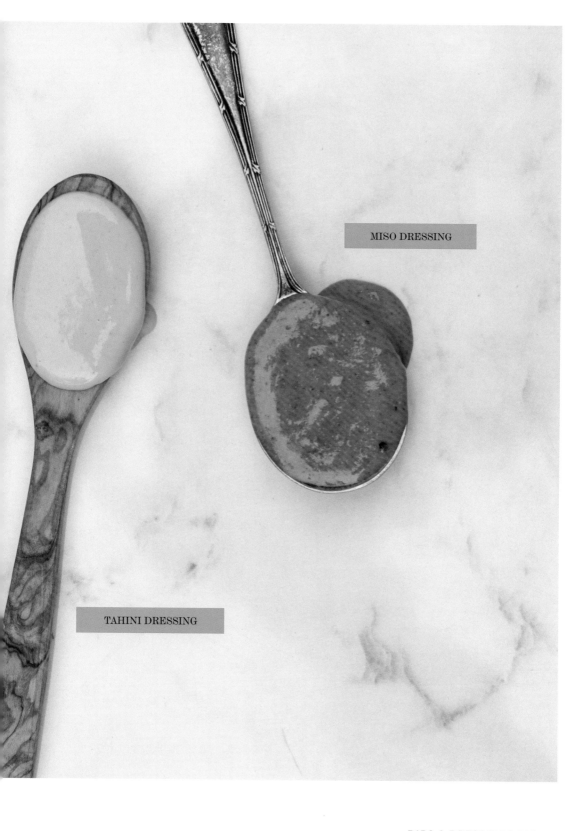

MISO DRESSING

TAHINI DRESSING

VEGAN MAYO

Vegan mayo makes everything a little tastier. Spread this on avocado toast, over cold potatoes for a quick potato salad or on a veggie burger. You can buy veganaise in health food stores, but if you're interested in making everything from scratch, here's how I do it.

Makes 7 oz (200g)

3½ oz (100g) sunflower seeds

1 tablespoon nutritional yeast

1 tablespoon fresh lemon juice

1 teaspoon raw apple cider vinegar

½ teaspoon maple or agave syrup

¼ teaspoon dry mustard

sea salt and freshly ground black
  pepper

approx. 5 fl oz 150ml grapeseed oil

1   Put the sunflower seeds in a small bowl, cover with cold filtered water and soak for at least 8 hours or ideally overnight. Drain and rinse, then pat them dry thoroughly with a clean tea towel or kitchen paper. (See the note on page 30 on soaking nuts.)

2   Put the soaked sunflower seeds in a high-powered blender with all the other ingredients except the grapeseed oil. Blitz to combine, then turn the blender down to a low speed and slowly drizzle in the oil. Season to taste with a little more salt and pepper if needed.

3   This will keep for up to three weeks in an airtight container in the fridge.

TIP: You can easily modify this by adding a little extra lemon juice or raw apple cider vinegar or perhaps some tamari (or soy sauce or coconut aminos) for a richer, more savoury flavour.

GARLIC MAYO

1   Put the sunflower seeds in a small bowl, cover with cold filtered water and soak for at least 8 hours or ideally overnight. Drain and rinse, then pat them dry thoroughly with a clean tea towel or kitchen paper. (See the note on page 30 on soaking nuts.)

2   Blend the sunflower seeds and add the lemon juice slowly so as to ensure the sauce blends as evenly as possible. Add the garlic and the nutritional yeast and the olive oil and a pinch of salt and pepper.

3   Taste it at this stage and before adding any more salt or pepper leave it to sit for a few moments. If it's too thick, add 1–2 teaspoons of warm filtered water to thin it to your preference.

4   It can be a classic case of needing more and more, then realising that you have added too much too quickly.

TIP: Try adding 1 teaspoon of Braggs liquid aminos or 1 teaspoon of miso paste – use white miso if possible to keep the lovely creamy colour. Brown miso will taste just as good but might not look as appetising!

There's a strong preconception that all vegan food is virtuous and people seem surprised that I don't want to exist solely on salad leaves. For me, eating well means having food that's satisfying on every level, and sometimes that means having a thick, creamy sauce and some fries to dip into it! I like to make at least one thick sauce like this every week, as a spoon or two transforms a simple salad, plate of roasted veg or a plain baked potato into something really tasty.

Makes 7 oz (200g)

3½ oz (100g) organic sunflower seeds

1 teaspoon lemon juice

2–4 garlic cloves, crushed, depending on how strong you want the garlic flavour to be

1 tablespoon nutritional yeast

approx. 5 fl oz (150ml) grapeseed oil

sea salt and freshly ground black pepper

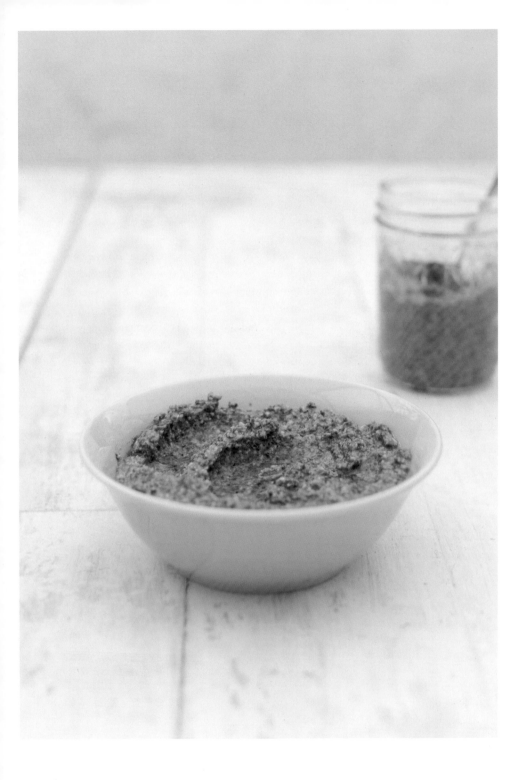

VEGAN PESTO

1   Put the basil, garlic, olive oil, lemon juice and nutritional yeast in a blender or food processor and pulse to combine. Add the pine nuts and pulse again until it's the consistency you like. I like it to have a chunky texture, so I blend for about 5 seconds and then it's ready.

2   Taste it before you add any seasoning and add only a little at a time. It's very easy to add more but you can't take it out if you add too much, so go slowly, taste again and suit your own palate.

3   The pesto is best made fresh but will hold in the fridge in an airtight container for a day or two.

This is so gorgeous and so versatile. Spread it on bread to enhance a simple sandwich or stir it into a bowl of pasta for a quick comforting meal. This is best made fresh, but thankfully it takes only 3 minutes to prep and blitz it up.

Makes 3⅓ fl oz (100ml)

1½ oz (40g) fresh basil, chopped

2 garlic cloves, crushed

6¾ fl oz (200ml) light olive oil

juice of ½ lemon

1 tablespoon nutritional yeast

3½ oz (100g) pine nuts

sea salt and freshly ground
   black pepper

AVOCADO AND SPINACH GARLIC AIOLI

Aquafaba is the water in a tin of chickpeas. I've thrown it down the drain countless times, but it turns out that the proteins in aquafaba mimic those in egg whites, so when used in the same proportions, they have the same effect. I wouldn't go substituting it for everything, but it works really well in this aioli. Adding the spinach and avocado gives it an amazing colour.

Makes 6¾ fl oz (200ml)

4 tablespoons aquafaba (see
   the intro)

1 teaspoon caster sugar

1 teaspoon raw apple cider vinegar

½ teaspoon Dijon mustard

4 teaspoons vegetable oil or any
   other flavourless oil

½ ripe avocado, peeled, stoned
   and sliced

a handful of baby spinach

2 garlic cloves, minced

1 tablespoon lemon juice

½ teaspoon fine sea salt

1 Put the aquafaba in a blender and pulse for about a minute. Add the sugar, vinegar and mustard and blend on high until everything is combined.

2 Keep the blender on high and trickle in the oil drop by drop. If you go too fast you'll ruin the whole thing, so be patient. If the oil is pooling on top, allow it to blend in before adding any more. It will suddenly turn creamy – at this stage, add the avocado, spinach, garlic, lemon juice and salt.

3 Store in an airtight container for up to two weeks in the fridge.

EPIC GUACAMOLE

1 To make a smooth guacamole, it works best to quickly process it in a blender or food processor. Pulse the avocados and lemon juice or vinegar together before adding in all the remaining ingredients and pulsing to combine.

2 If you are mashing by hand to make a guacamole with a little more texture, start by breaking down the avocado and blending with the lemon juice or vinegar before folding in the remaining ingredients.

TIP: If you want this to be extra sharp, add 1 teaspoon of lemon zest.

Frozen avocados are a recent addition to supermarket shelves, and while they are great for smoothies, they definitely don't work well for guacamole. The avocado is the star here, and frozen ones don't blend as well with the other ingredients as fresh avocados do.

Buying avocados is such a tricky business, but here's a little tip: when shopping, pull off the little tip at the top. If the avocado feels firm but the little bit of flesh showing under the tip is brown, it's gone too far. You want a firm texture and that lovely light green colour. I always recommend buying one extra, just in case, so that your breakfast or snack won't be ruined if the avocado gods aren't on your side with your first try!

Serves 2

2 ripe avocados, peeled, stoned and
   flesh scooped out
1 tablespoon lemon juice or raw apple
   cider vinegar
4 cherry tomatoes, finely chopped
2 garlic cloves, crushed
a pinch of paprika or chilli powder
   (if you like a little heat)
sea salt and freshly ground
   black pepper

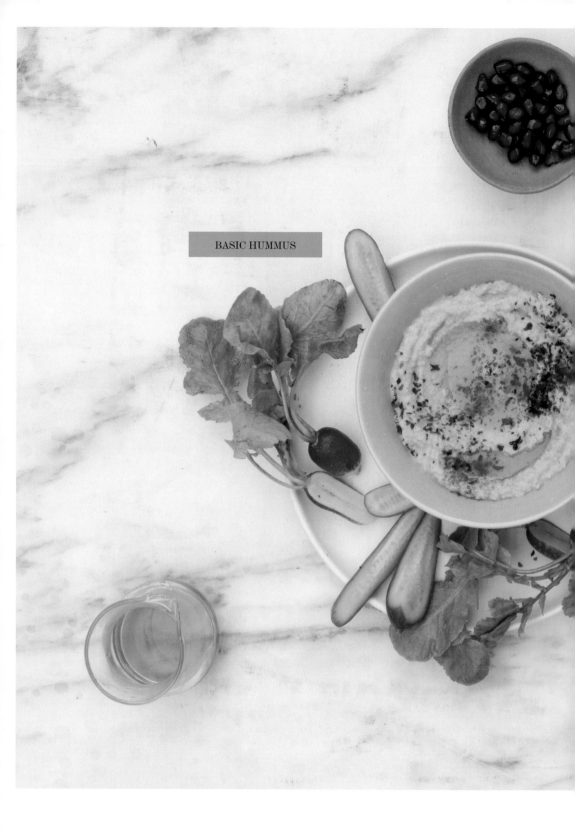

BASIC HUMMUS

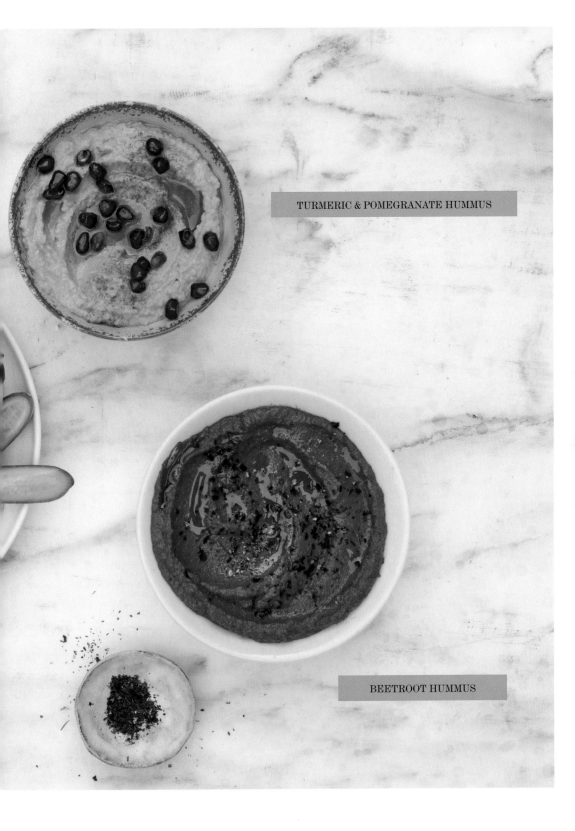

TURMERIC & POMEGRANATE HUMMUS

BEETROOT HUMMUS

LEMON AND GARLIC HUMMUS

Hummus is readily available now to buy in shops, but it's so simple to make your own.

Makes 1¾ lb (800g)

2 x 14 oz (400g) tins of chickpeas, drained and rinsed

1 lemon, peeled, chopped and seeds removed

3 garlic cloves, peeled and finely sliced

4 tablespoons olive oil, plus extra to serve

3 tablespoons filtered water

2 heaped tablespoons tahini

2 teaspoons ground cumin

sea salt and freshly ground black pepper

1 Put all the ingredients in a food processor and blend until smooth. Drizzle in a little more water if needed to get your desired consistency. The stronger your food processor is, the smoother and creamier the hummus will be. Season to taste with salt and pepper.

2 Serve with a drizzle of olive oil on top. Store in an airtight container in the fridge for up to a week.

TIP: If you want to use dried chickpeas that you've soaked and boiled yourself, you'll need approx. 1 lb (450g) cooked chickpeas.

I like to add a whole lemon as there is so much goodness and flavour in the pith, but if you don't want your hummus to be too sharp, add only half the lemon, taste it and add more if needed.

BEETROOT HUMMUS

1   Put the chickpeas, lemon, garlic, olive oil, water, tahini and cumin in a food processor and blend until smooth. Drizzle in a little more water if needed to get your desired consistency. The stronger your food processor is, the smoother and creamier the hummus will be. Season to taste with salt and pepper.

2   Add the beetroot piece by piece, blending after each addition, tasting until you're happy with the flavour.

3   Serve with a drizzle of olive oil and a pinch of dulse on top (if using). Store in an airtight container in the fridge for up to a week.

TIP: If you want to use dried chickpeas that you've soaked and boiled yourself, you'll need approx. 1 lb (450g) cooked chickpeas.

I like to add a whole lemon as there is so much goodness and flavour in the pith, but if you don't want your hummus to be too sharp, then add only half the lemon, taste it and add more if liked.

I don't really like beetroot by itself, but I love it blended into smoothies and juices or, in this case, hummus. This really shows how easy it is to customise your hummus. For example, you can add leftover roasted veggies to the mix – carrots will add sweetness and roasted garlic works well too. The colour of this beetroot hummus will blow your mind!

Makes 1¾ lb (800g)

2 x 14 oz (400g) tins of chickpeas, drained and rinsed

1 lemon, peeled, chopped and seeds removed

3 garlic cloves, peeled and finely sliced

4 tablespoons olive oil, plus extra to serve

3 tablespoons filtered water

2 heaped tablespoons tahini

2 teaspoons ground cumin

sea salt and freshly ground black pepper

1–2 cooked beetroots, chopped

milled dulse seaweed, to garnish (optional)

TURMERIC AND POMEGRANATE HUMMUS

Hummus is a great canvas for different flavours and something so simple can easily become really special with a few ingredients. This is a beautiful starter served in a big bowl with a drizzle of olive oil on top and some chunky sourdough bread to dip in it.

Makes 1¾ lb (800g)

2 x 14 oz (400g) tins of chickpeas, drained and rinsed

1 lemon, peeled, chopped and seeds removed

3 garlic cloves, peeled and finely sliced

4 tablespoons olive oil, plus extra to serve

3 tablespoons filtered water

2 heaped tablespoons tahini

2 teaspoons ground cumin

1 teaspoon ground turmeric

sea salt and freshly ground black pepper

1 tablespoon pomegranate seeds

1   Put the chickpeas, lemon, garlic, olive oil, water, tahini, cumin and turmeric in a food processor and blend until smooth. Drizzle in a little more water if needed to get your desired consistency. The stronger your food processor is, the smoother and creamier the hummus will be. Season to taste with salt and pepper, then fold in the pomegranate seeds.

2   Serve with a drizzle of olive oil on top. Store in an airtight container in the fridge for up to a week.

TIP: If you want to use dried chickpeas that you've soaked and boiled yourself, you'll need approx. 1 lb (450g) cooked chickpeas.

I like to add a whole lemon as there is so much goodness and flavour in the pith, but if you don't want your hummus to be too sharp, then add only half the lemon, taste it and add more if liked.

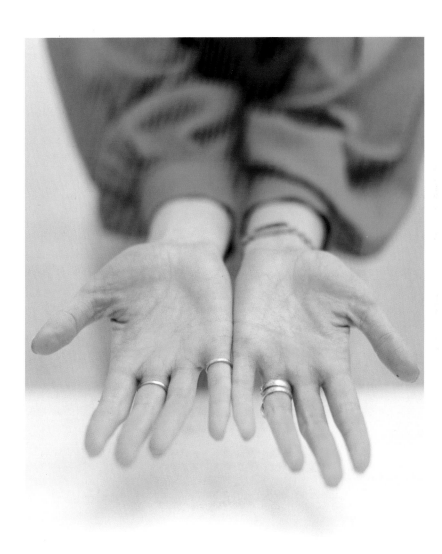

Creating my own crackers first came about from wondering what to do with leftover almond milk pulp. Gradually, as my confidence grew, I began to create my own breads using all the nuts and seeds I love. I like nutrient-dense food, and if you make the All-Day Bread you will see it lives up to its name – it will keep you going all day long!

BREADS & CRACKERS

ALL-DAY BREAD

Makes 1 loaf

DRY INGREDIENTS:

5⅔ oz (160g) hulled sunflower seeds

2¼ oz (65g) hulled pumpkin seeds

3¼ oz (90g) almonds

8¼ oz (235g) rolled oats

4¼ oz (140g) flaxseeds

⅘ oz (25g) psyllium seed husks (see the tips)

⅘ oz (25g) chia seeds

1 teaspoon fine sea salt

WET INGREDIENTS:

2⅔ cup (625ml) filtered water

1½ oz (40g) maple or agave syrup or approx. 2 oz (55g) date syrup

approx. 2 oz (55g) olive or coconut oil, plus extra for greasing

1 Preheat the oven to 350°F (180°C). Grease a 2lb loaf tin with a little olive or coconut oil or line it with a paper liner or non-stick baking paper.

2 Spread the sunflower and pumpkin seeds on a baking tray and put the almonds on a separate tray. Toast in the oven for about 15 minutes, stirring halfway through, until they start to brown. Allow to cool and turn off the oven. Coarsely chop the almonds.

3 Put all the dry ingredients, including the toasted seeds, into a large bowl and mix to combine. Whisk together the wet ingredients in a jug, then pour them into the bowl with the dry ingredients. Mix up the 'dough' really well. Don't be afraid to use your hands to knead away your stress – it will actually make the bread even better!

4 Scoop the dough into the prepared loaf tin and smooth out the top. Bang the tin down on the counter a few times to ensure there are no air bubbles. If you have any seeds left over, you can decorate the top with them or even spell out your initials if you like! Put in the refrigerator and leave it for several hours, or ideally overnight.

5 When you're ready to bake, remove the bread from the fridge and let it come to room temperature.

6 Put a rack in the middle of the oven and preheat it to 400°F (200°C).

7 Bake the bread for about 1 hour, then take it out and gently remove the loaf from the pan. Let it cool on a wire rack for at least 2 hours. They say good things come to those who wait and this bread involves a lot of waiting, but it will live up to your expectations. Slice it thinly and serve toasted. This lasts for up to a week in an airtight container stored in the fridge.

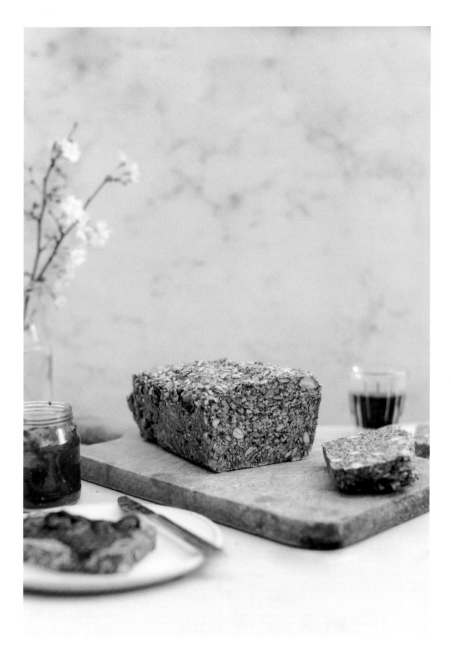

TIPS: The binding agent here is psyllium seed husks and they are essential. You can find them in health food stores or online.

If you're starting from scratch with all the ingredients it will seem like a costly shop, but bear in mind that you should have enough of most of the ingredients to make this at least twice, and in the case of the psyllium husks there should be enough in one container to make several loaves.

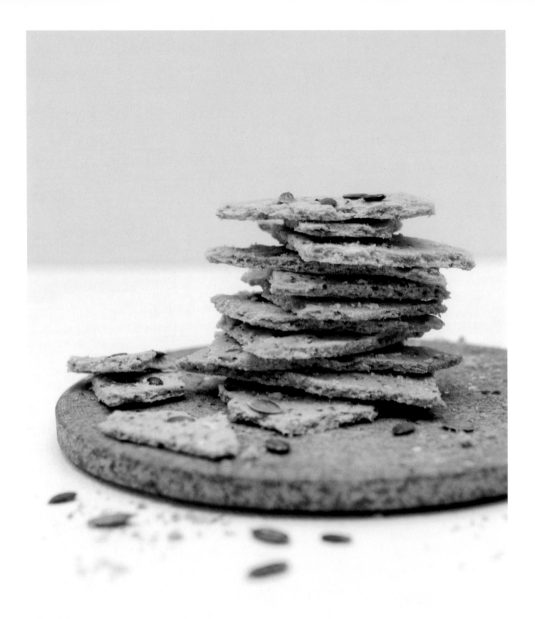

TIPS: If you don't have or can't find shop-bought almond flour, you can grind whole almonds to a fine flour in a high-powered blender or food processor, but don't over-process them or they'll release their oils, which you don't want.

You can find brown rice flour in health food shops or online.

ANYTHING GOES CRACKERS

1 Preheat the oven to 350°F (180°C). Line a baking tray with non-stick baking paper, then lightly brush the paper with a little olive oil.

2 Put all the dry ingredients in a large mixing bowl and mix to combine (omit the pumpkin seeds if you'd rather scatter them on top of the crackers). Whisk together the oil and water in a jug, then pour into the dry ingredients and mix well with a spoon or your hands.

3 Put the dough on the lined baking tray. Put another piece of baking paper on top of the dough and roll it out until it's about ¼" (6mm) thick. Remove the top piece of baking paper. Scatter over the pumpkin seeds if you've saved them.

4 Use a pizza cutter or knife to score the dough lightly into the shape and size you want your crackers to be. These scored lines will form the breaking point when the crackers are finished. I just break up the crackers by hand without scoring the dough, as I'm not looking for symmetry, so do what you like best.

5 Bake in the oven for 20–25 minutes, until the middle of the cracker is firm to touch with the back of a spoon. The thicker they are, the longer they will take to bake. Likewise, if you have made them very thin they will cook very quickly, so you have to trust your judgement here. Remove from the oven and allow to cool on the tray for at least 1 hour before you break them up.

6 These will keep in an airtight container for up to a week. If they need to be crisped up, put them back in a hot oven for a few minutes.

The name of these crackers says it all! I rarely have bread in the house, as it's something I haven't mastered yet, but I love crackers. These are a great way to use up all your old packets of seeds and nuts.

Makes 18 crackers

1 lb 2 oz (500g) almond flour

3½ oz (100g) brown rice flour

1½ oz (40g) pumpkin seeds

2 tablespoons milled chia seeds

1 tablespoon nutritional yeast

1 teaspoon dried herbes de Provence
   or mixed herbs

¼ teaspoon garlic powder

a pinch of baking soda

3⅓ fl oz (100ml) olive oil, plus extra for
   greasing

2 fl oz (60ml) filtered water

ALMOND CRACKERS

Once I started to make almond milk regularly I wanted to find inventive ways to use the leftover pulp, so I developed these savoury crackers and now I prefer them to most store-bought ones. You can adjust the flavour to your preferences, making them more savoury or even injecting a little spice with some chilli powder or paprika. This is a simple neutral recipe that works well with whatever dip or hummus you serve with the crackers.

Makes 10 crackers

1 tablespoon chia seeds

1 tablespoon filtered water

3½ oz (100g) wet almond pulp (see the intro)

1 garlic clove, minced

2 tablespoons olive oil, plus extra for greasing

1 tablespoon ground flaxseeds (see the tip)

½ teaspoon onion powder

½ teaspoon ground cumin

1   Preheat the oven to 350°F (170°C). Line a baking tray with non-stick baking paper and brush the paper lightly with a little olive oil. If you're using a dehydrator, have your silicone sheet close to hand.

2   Put the chia seeds in a small bowl with the tablespoon of water. Set aside for about 10 minutes to allow the seeds to gel.

3   Put all the ingredients, including the soaked chia seeds, in a large bowl. Mix together with a spoon, then use your hands to ensure everything is thoroughly blended. The more you mix this, the better your crackers will stick together without flaking apart, so spend at least 2 minutes kneading the mixture before spreading it out on the lined tray or silicone sheet. Press it down with a spatula or your hands into an even layer, but don't spread it too thinly.

4   Use a pizza cutter or knife to score the dough lightly into the shape and size you want your crackers to be. These scored lines will form the breaking point when the crackers are finished. I just break up the crackers by hand without scoring the dough, as I'm not looking for symmetry, so do what you like best.

5   Bake in the oven for 30–40 minutes, until firm to touch, or dehydrate overnight. The thicker they are, the longer they will take to bake. Likewise, if you have made them very thin they will cook very quickly, so you have to trust your judgement here. Remove from the oven and allow to cool on the tray for at least 1 hour before you break them up.

6   Store in an airtight container for up to a week. If they need to be crisped up, put them back in a hot oven for a few minutes.

TIPS: You need to use up almond pulp quickly. Don't leave it on your counter intending to do something with it later, as it will go off after just one day.

If you don't have ground flaxseeds, just grind whole ones in a high-powered blender or coffee grinder.

If you want a really smooth texture you could blend everything together in a food processor, but your hands are the best mixing tool for these, as there's a bit of squelching involved, and the more thoroughly mixed they are, the firmer your crackers will be.

It's amazing that traditions that have been used for centuries to preserve food have been forgotten, but thankfully there is now a revival happening and Kombucha is widely available. Making your own is easier than you might think, and from a health perspective, filling your plate with live, nutritious ferments is definitely a move in the right direction.

FERMENTATION

KOMBUCHA

One of the first cooking courses I did was a 12-week course called Raw Food Mastery where we learned about sprouting, fermentation, raw chocolate, sauerkraut, kimchi and medicinal teas. Darren, our teacher, would put jugs of his powerfully strong kombucha on the table for us to help ourselves. Soon I was set up at home with my scoby and kefir grains and a newfound passion for live foods and a curiosity to experiment.

You can buy a scoby online, but if you have a friend who makes kombucha, I'm sure they will be happy to share, as they multiply quickly if you are fermenting regularly. The word scoby is actually an acronym that stands for symbiotic culture of bacteria and yeast. A scoby is the living home for the bacteria and yeast that transform sweet tea into tangy, fizzy, live kombucha.

You'll need 2 x 4¼-cup (1-litre) mason jars for this.

Makes 4¼ cups (1 litre)

4¼ cup (1 litre) filtered water
4 tea bags (see the tips)
approx. 2 oz (60g) organic sugar
1 kombucha scoby

1   Wash a 8½-cup (2-litre or larger) mason jar in hot soapy water and make sure you rinse it well.
2   Boil the water, then pour it into the jar and add the tea bags to brew a strong tea. Leave it to stand for at least 1 hour, until cooled. Stir in the sugar with a clean wooden spoon. When cooled to below 100°F (37°C) (lukewarm), add the scoby.
3   Leave the lid open slightly to expose the kombucha to the air, but cover the jar with a clean tea towel or muslin cloth secured with an elastic band to stop dust or flies from getting in. Leave the jar in a warm place away from direct sunlight for one week.
4   After a week, taste it to see if you're happy with the flavour. The bacteria in the scoby eat the sugar, so you know it's ready when it's not too sweet. I like mine after 10 days. If you leave it much longer than that, it can be too tart.
5   Pour the kombucha into another clean 4¼-cup (1-litre) mason jar for the second ferment. I always leave about 1" (2.5cm) worth of kombucha in the base of the original jar as the starter for my next brew (see the tips). I like to add some fruit to flavour the second ferment – try raspberry and lemon (page 260) or lime and ginger (page 261) – but you can leave it plain if you prefer.
6   Close this jar firmly to allow the carbonation (fizziness) to build up. After 24 hours, you need to 'burp' the jar by opening it to allow some of the pressure to escape. Repeat this every day. After three days, it will be nicely carbonated and ready to drink. At this point, store the kombucha in the fridge to stop the fermentation and drink within one month.

TIPS: I've experimented with different black teas, but I prefer kombucha made with organic green tea. Play around to see what you like best.

I use a large mason jar with a tap at the bottom so that when the kombucha is ready, it's easy to pour out. Using the continuous brew method, I add my next batch of tea straight into the first mason jar. There's no need to clean the jar in between batches – in fact, this will interfere with the beneficial environment you've created for fermentation to take place.

KOMBUCHA WITH RASPBERRY AND LEMON

When flavouring kombucha you're dealing with completely natural ingredients that differ every time you use them, so your kombucha will taste slightly different every time. That said, there are a few simple guidelines to follow when flavouring kombucha and putting it through a second ferment. As a general rule, if you're flavouring the kombucha with fresh, frozen or dried fruit, start with 15% fruit and 85% kombucha. If you're flavouring it with juice, start with 10% juice and 90% kombucha.

Makes enough for 8 x 4¼-cup (1-litre) bottles

3½ oz (100g) fresh or frozen raspberries
1 tablespoon organic sugar
juice of 4 lemons

1 Combine the raspberries, sugar and lemon juice in a high-powered blender, then sieve to remove the raspberry seeds.
2 Pour 1 tablespoon of this purée into a 4¼-cup (1-litre) bottle of kombucha that's ready for its second ferment, leaving about 2" (5cm) of space clear at the top of the bottle to allow for the extra carbonation that will build up. Pour the rest of the purée into 1 tablespoon portions in an ice cube and freeze, making your next ferment really convenient.
3 Close the jar firmly to allow the carbonation (fizziness) to build up. After 24 hours, you need to 'burp' the jar by opening it to allow some of the pressure to escape. Burp the jar the next day too. After two days, it will be nicely carbonated and ready to drink. At this point, store the kombucha in the fridge to stop the fermentation and drink within one month.

TIPS: It works best to blend the berries and lemon juice as that makes it easier for the kombucha to access the natural sugars, but you could add the whole berries and lemon juice directly to the kombucha for its second ferment. In that case, add six berries and a 1" (2.5cm) wedge of peeled lemon per litre.

You must ensure there is absolutely no mould or dirt on the berries, as this will disrupt the fermentation process.

KOMBUCHA WITH LIME AND GINGER

1 Put the lime and ginger pieces and the sugar directly in the kombucha when it's ready for its second ferment, leaving about 2" (5cm) of space clear at the top of the bottle to allow for the extra carbonation that will build up. Close the jar firmly.

2 After 24 hours, you need to 'burp' the jar by opening it to allow some of the pressure to escape. Burp the jar the next day too. After two days, it will be nicely carbonated and ready to drink. At this point, store the kombucha in the fridge to stop the fermentation and drink within one month.

TIP: You'll get the best flavour by juicing the lime and ginger before you put it into your kombucha.

Ginger works so well in kombucha and the sharpness of the lime gives it a nice tang. This is the kind of thing I crave when I haven't had it for a while.

Makes enough for 4¼ cups (1 litre) of kombucha

½ lime, peeled and sliced

1 x 2" (5cm) piece of fresh ginger, peeled and chopped

1 teaspoon organic sugar

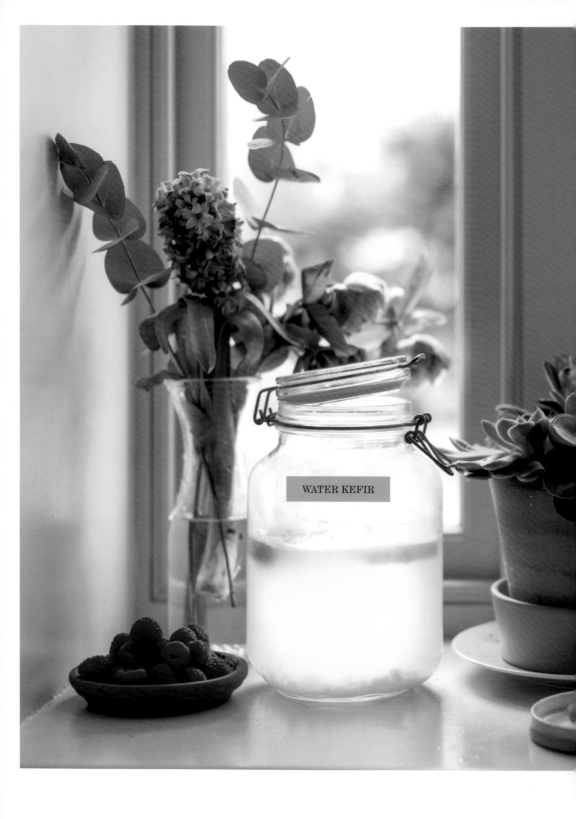

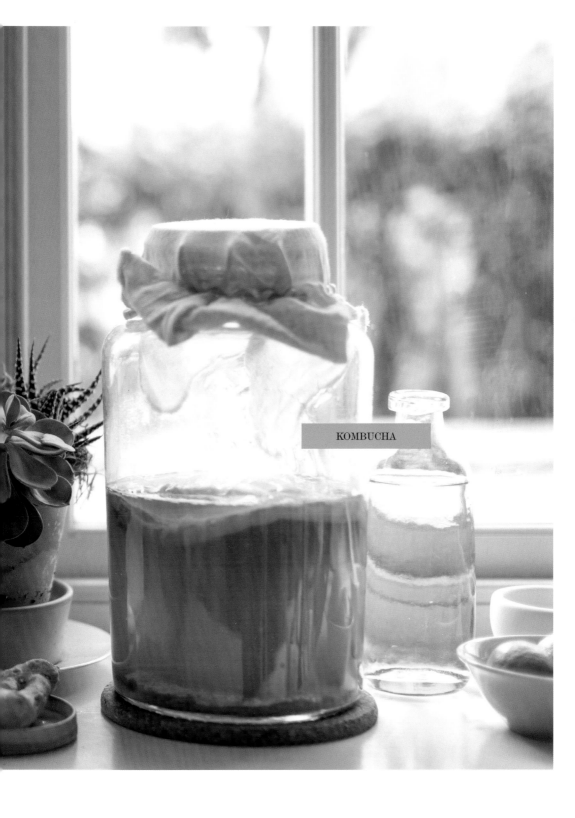

KOMBUCHA

WATER KEFIR

Water kefir is like kombucha's less powerful sibling, with a lighter flavour. I'm always a bit cynical when people say healthy things are just like something that's not so healthy, but when made right, water kefir is similar to a soft drink and is really refreshing.

You'll need 2 x 4¼-cup (1-litre) mason jars for this.

Makes 4¼ cups (1 litre)

1¾ oz (50g) caster sugar, plus 1 teaspoon if doing a second ferment

4¼ cup (1 litre) filtered boiled water, cooled to room temperature, plus extra to dissolve the sugar

2 dried unsulphured figs

1 organic unwaxed lemon, scrubbed and cut in half (if your lemon isn't organic or unwaxed, cut off the peel)

4 tablespoons water kefir grains

1 Dissolve the 1¾ oz (50g) of sugar in a small cup of just-boiled water and allow to cool. Pour into a sterilised 4¼-cup (1-litre) mason jar (see the note on page 30 on how to sterilise jars) and top up with the litre of cooled boiled water. Add the figs, lemon and kefir grains.

2 Cover the jar with a clean muslin cloth secured with an elastic band and leave to ferment for two or three days in a warm place away from draughts. Strain it through a non-reactive fine-mesh strainer (see the tips) into a clean 4¼-cup (1-litre) bottle. Discard the spent lemon and figs, but reserve the water kefir grains, which can be immediately reused or stored in the fridge for up to a week in a jar of filtered water in which you've dissolved 1 tablespoon of organic sugar.

3 You can drink the kefir now and store it in the fridge for up to two months, but to do a second ferment, add 1 teaspoon of sugar to the jar, then top up with the kefir, leaving 1" (2.5cm) of head room clear at the top of the jar. (Alternatively, make a pineapple and lemon version – see the tips.) I usually leave it to ferment again for one or two days. You need to 'burp' the jar every morning by opening it to allow some of the pressure from the carbonation to escape, otherwise your jar might explode!

4 At this point, transfer the water kefir to the fridge and don't open it for three days to allow the bubbles to set. Open carefully over a sink, as the liquid in the bottle is under pressure from the carbonation, and when you release the bottle's seal the water kefir may fizz and foam.

5 Drink this on its own or use it in smoothies or cashew yogurt (page 58) for an immediate probiotic boost.

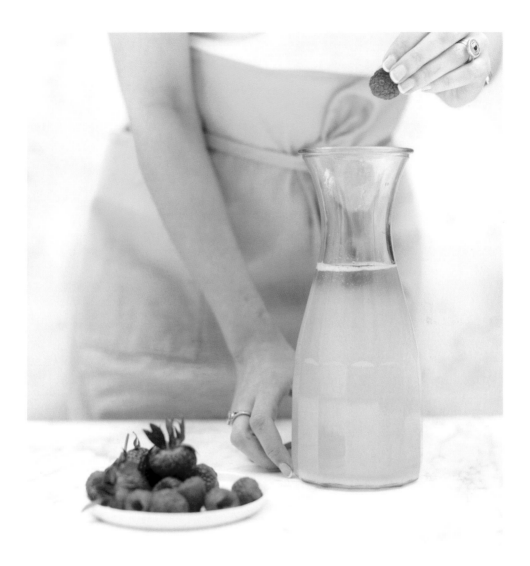

TIPS: Only use non-reactive utensils with kefir grains. The grains are acidic, so they react with metals. If you'll be making kefir regularly, invest in a set of plastic or stainless steel measuring spoons and a plastic fine-mesh sieve.

When you first purchase your kefir grains you might not have the 4 tablespoons called for in this recipe, but don't worry – they will naturally grow with every batch you make. Once the kefir grains start to multiply – and they will! – you can give them away to friends. Just make sure you always keep at least 4 tablespoons to start a fresh batch.

To make a pineapple and lemon water kefir, add 1 tablespoon of lemon juice and a 1" (2.5cm) wedge of pineapple or 1 tablespoon of pineapple juice to your kefir for its second ferment.

COCONUT WATER KEFIR

Coconut water kefir is very easy and you don't need to worry so much about ratios.

Makes 4¼ cups (1 litre)

4¼ cup (1 litre) coconut water
4 tablespoons water kefir grains

1   Simply pour the coconut water into a sterilised 4¼-cup (1-litre) jar (see the note on page 30 on how to sterilise jars) and add your kefir grains. Cover the jar with a muslin cloth secured with an elastic band and leave to ferment for at least 24 hours in a warm place away from draughts.

2   Strain it though a plastic fine-mesh sieve into a clean 4¼-cup (1-litre) bottle and store in the fridge. Flavour it however you like or use it in smoothies or to make coconut yogurt (see pages 52–57).

TIPS: Only use non-reactive utensils with kefir grains. The grains are acidic, so they react with metals. If you'll be making kefir regularly, invest in a set of plastic or stainless steel measuring spoons and a plastic fine-mesh sieve.

Once the kefir grains start to multiply – and they will! – you can give them away to friends. Just make sure you keep at least 4 tablespoons to start a fresh batch.

KIMCHI

1 Cut the cabbage lengthwise into quarters and remove the core. Cut each quarter across into 2" (5cm)-wide strips. Put the cabbage in a large bowl and sprinkle with salt. Massage the salt into the cabbage until it starts to soften a bit, then add enough filtered water to cover the cabbage. Put a plate on top and weigh it down with something heavy, like a tin of beans. Allow to stand for 1–2 hours.

2 Drain and rinse the cabbage and leave to stand until it's as dry as possible, gently squeezing to remove as much of the water as you can.

3 Meanwhile, put all the sauce ingredients in a high-powered blender and blitz to combine.

4 Put the cabbage, daikon, carrots, shallot and probiotics in a large mixing bowl and toss together, then pour the sauce over the vegetables. Wearing gloves, as the gochugaru will stain your hands and sting badly if you have any cuts, massage the sauce into the vegetables.

5 Transfer to a sterilised 4¼-cup (1-litre) mason jar (see the note on page 30 on how to sterilise jars), pressing down on the veg until the brine rises up to cover them. Seal the jar and allow it to ferment at room temperature for up to five days. Check it daily and press the vegetables down with the back of a clean spoon to ensure they are always submerged.

6 Taste it daily, and when it's to your liking, transfer the jar to the fridge. You may see bubbles inside the jar and brine may seep out of the lid, so put a bowl or plate under the jar to help catch any overflow.

Fermented foods are an easy addition to any meal and you will be amazed at how reasonable they are to make yourself compared to buying them.
Makes 1¾ lb (800g)

14 oz (400g) Chinese cabbage (approx. ½ head)
fine sea salt
cold filtered water
7 oz (200g) daikon radish, finely chopped
2 large carrots, finely chopped
1 shallot, finely chopped
1 probiotic capsule, split open

FOR THE SAUCE:
3 garlic cloves, minced (approx. ¾ oz [20g])
1 shallot, finely chopped
¾ oz (20g) fresh ginger, peeled and finely chopped
2 tablespoons tamari, soy sauce or coconut aminos
1 tablespoon filtered water
1 tablespoon olive oil
1½ teaspoons miso paste
1 heaped teaspoon gochugaru (Korean red pepper powder)
sea salt and freshly ground black pepper

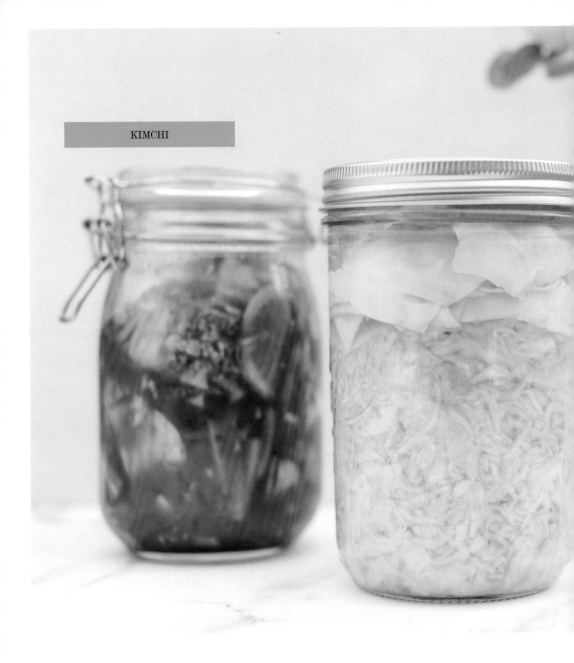

KIMCHI

TIPS: Always make sure that the brine is covering the kimchi when storing it in the fridge, otherwise it can go mouldy.

If you have a mandoline or a slicing attachment on your food processor, use it to get lovely thin slices of carrot and radish.

You can find the Korean red pepper in Asian markets or online.

A word of caution: too much garlic can make the kimchi bitter and too much ginger can make it sticky. As for the gochugaru, adjust the amount to your liking. Kimchi can be mild or fiery – it's your choice.

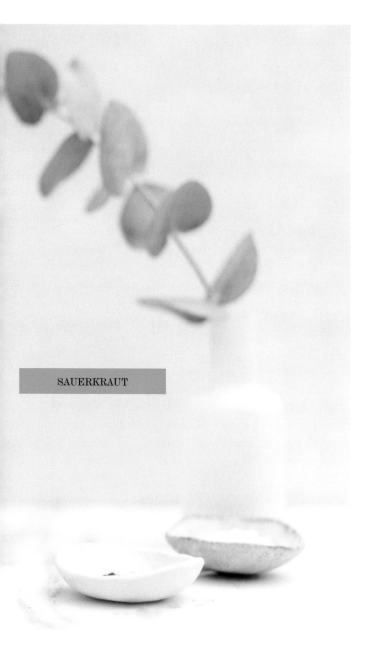

SAUERKRAUT

SAUERKRAUT

Sauerkraut is the perfect introduction to fermentation, as it's so easy to make. It's a delicious addition to veggie burgers, Buddha bowls and salads. Sauerkraut contains a lot of the same healthy probiotics as a bowl of yogurt.

Makes a 4¼-cup (1-litre) jar

2 heads of green cabbage, ideally
   organic
1 tablespoon Himalayan pink salt

1 Take off a few of the big outer leaves from the cabbage and set aside to use at the end.

2 Shred the cabbage with a mandoline or in a food processor fitted with a slicing attachment and put it in a large bowl. Rinse it well and drain as much of the water off as possible before sprinkling over the salt. Leave it for a few minutes to allow the salt to start pulling the water from the cabbage. Using your hands, massage the salt into the cabbage to help it release its water until there is enough juice to submerge all the cabbage under it.

3 Transfer to a sterilised 4¼-cup (1-litre) mason jar (see the note on page 30 on how to sterilise jars) and really push it down to compress and submerge the cabbage under the brine. Put some of the large outer leaves on top and press them down tightly. Don't seal the lid, but put a clean muslin cloth on top, secured with a rubber band, to stop any dust or flies getting into it.

4 Store your jar away from direct sunlight at room temperature for up to seven days to allow it to ferment. Check it daily and press it down if the cabbage is floating above the liquid. Start tasting it after three days – when the sauerkraut tastes good to you, screw on the lid and refrigerate it. There's no hard-and-fast rule for when the sauerkraut is done. You can allow it to continue fermenting for 10 days or even longer – go by how it tastes.

5   During the fermenting stage you may see
bubbles coming up through the cabbage, foam
on the top or white scum. These are all signs of
a healthy fermentation process. The scum can be
skimmed off the top either during fermentation
or before refrigerating. If you see any mould, skim
it off immediately and make sure your cabbage is
fully submerged under the brine. Don't eat any
mouldy parts close to the surface, but the rest of the
sauerkraut is fine.

6   Sauerkraut is a fermented food, so it will keep
safely for at least two months in the fridge.

I use quite a lot of nut butters in my recipes and usually make my own. Once you have a strong food processor you will be amazed by how quickly you can start whipping them up. Whether you want a savoury almond butter, a gorgeous chia jam or a chocolate spread that you'll want to eat straight from the jar, it's all in here.

NUT BUTTERS & JAMS

MIXED NUT BUTTER WITH HIMALAYAN PINK SALT

Whether it's to thicken a smoothie, dollop on top of yogurt or to use in a salad or satay dressing, this is an essential staple in my kitchen that I use nearly every day.

Makes 14 oz (400g)

14 oz (400g) almonds, cashews, macadamia and/or Brazil nuts
½ teaspoon Himalayan pink salt
1 teaspoon melted coconut oil, if necessary

1 Preheat the oven to 300°F (150°C).

2 Spread the nuts out on a baking tray and toast them in the oven for about 8 minutes, until golden. Keep an eye on them to make sure they don't burn. You can also toast them in a hot dry pan, but you'll need to keep stirring them to make sure they toast evenly. Don't try to skip this step unless you have an extremely strong food processor, as you'll end up with almond meal that won't ever break down, resulting in a waste of costly ingredients and a lot of frustration.

3 Put the toasted nuts in a strong food processor and blend for up to 10 minutes, until a creamy paste is formed. You might need to stop and use a spatula to scrape down the sides and push down any nuts that get stuck.

4 If it's still not breaking down after 10 minutes, add the teaspoon of coconut oil through the funnel to loosen it while the motor is still running. If you're using oiler nuts, like macadamias, this might not be required. Unless it really needs it, don't add any more coconut oil, as it can leave an oily film on top of your nut butter when it settles. Allow it to blend for another few minutes and a smooth nut butter should form.

5 Scoop the nut butter into a small sterilised jar with a tight-sealing lid (see the note on page 30 on how to sterilise jars). Store in the fridge for up to one month (see the note on nut butter shelf life on page 31).

TIPS: Adding chia or flaxseeds makes your nut butter a little healthier and more filling and it also adds a little crunch to the texture.

Nuts are pricey, so keep an eye out for in-store offers but check the sell-by date, as nuts should have a long shelf life. Even though buying a approx. 2¼ lb (kilo) of cashews might seem like a lot at the time, you'll be surprised how quickly you use them. Check out shops online too, but be careful, as the shipping costs can increase the final price significantly. Sometimes sites do sales with free shipping, so sign up for alerts on your favourite sites. Asian markets that sell to catering outlets and restaurants always have a great selection of nuts as well and are often a little more reasonably priced. Be sure to stock up on rice, tamari and spices while you're there!

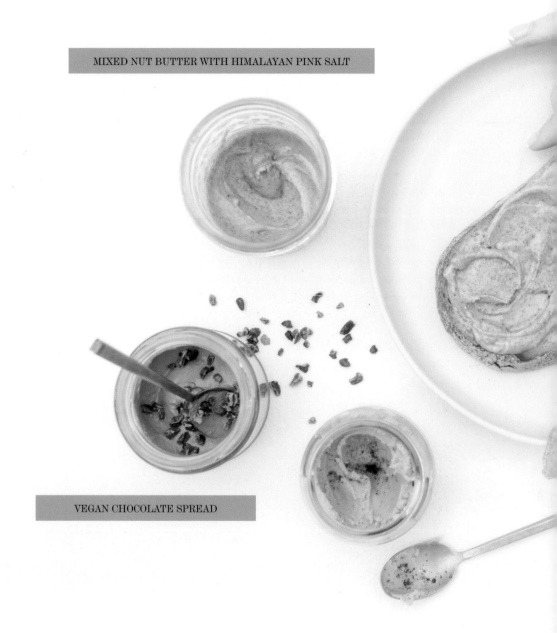

MIXED NUT BUTTER WITH HIMALAYAN PINK SALT

VEGAN CHOCOLATE SPREAD

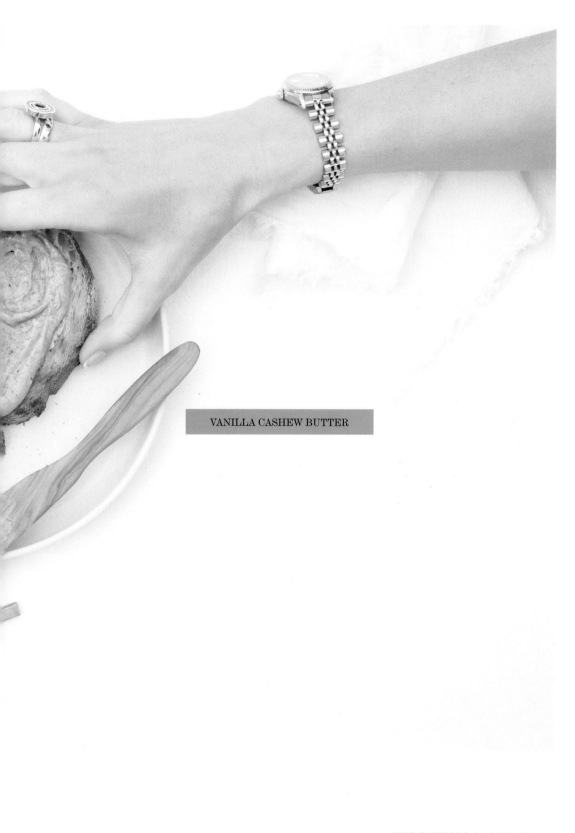

VANILLA CASHEW BUTTER

VANILLA CASHEW BUTTER

I was shopping in a health food store one day when I came across vanilla powder. It smelled so sweet and delicious that I wanted to find a way to use it so that I could have a little of that taste as often as possible. It can be quite expensive, but it totally changes the flavour of what you are making to something really special. A few vanilla pods will have the same effect if you can't find the powder.

When I first made this I finally understood how people can eat jars of nut butter by the spoonful straight from the jar. Dipping a square of dark chocolate into it or spreading some onto fresh summer strawberries is a gorgeous combination.

Makes 14 oz (400g)

14 oz (400g) cashew nuts

4 Medjool dates, pitted and sliced

1 heaped teaspoon vanilla powder
   or 3 vanilla pods, cut in half
   lengthways and seeds scraped out

1 teaspoon melted coconut oil, if
   necessary

1 Preheat the oven to 300°F (150°C).

2 Spread the cashews out on a baking tray and toast them in the oven for about 8 minutes, until golden. Keep an eye on them to make sure they don't burn.

3 Put the toasted nuts in a strong food processor and blend for up to 10 minutes, until a creamy paste is formed. You might need to stop and use a spatula to scrape down the sides and push down any nuts that get stuck.

4 With the motor still running, slowly add the chopped dates through the funnel along with the vanilla powder. If it forms a ball, add the teaspoon of coconut oil through the funnel with the motor still running to loosen it. Allow it to blend for another few minutes and a smooth nut butter should form. Unless it really needs it, don't add any more coconut oil, as it can leave an oily film on top of your nut butter when it settles.

5 Scoop the nut butter into a small sterilised jar with a tight-sealing lid (see the note on page 30 on how to sterilise jars). Store in the fridge for up to one month (see the note on nut butter shelf life on page 31).

TIP: Don't forget to take out the stones from the dates! And don't be tempted to soak them, as the water will change the consistency of the nut butter. If you can't get Medjool dates, 4 tablespoons of agave syrup will also work.

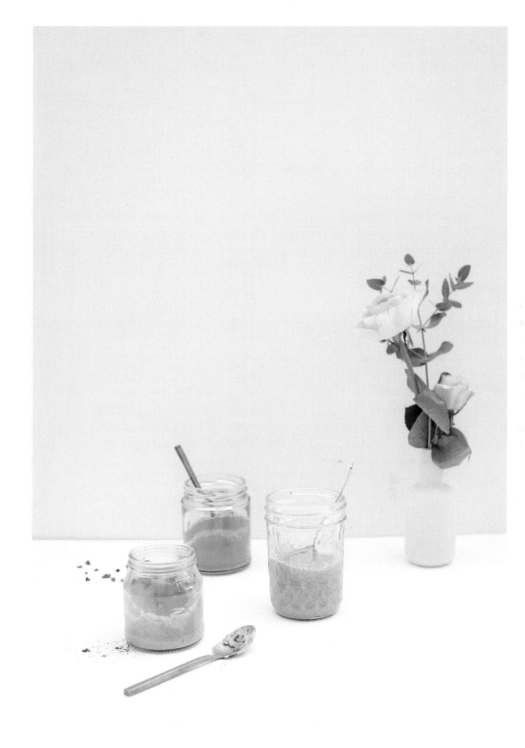

VEGAN CHOCOLATE SPREAD

This is a really simple sweet treat. I love it on fresh berries with some chopped nuts on top. It's also amazing on dairy-free ice cream. It takes a bit of effort and you need a high-powered blender to get it super smooth but it's well worth it.

Makes 1 small jar

7 oz (200g) hazelnuts

1¾ oz (50g) cacao butter or coconut oil

4 tablespoons of agave or maple syrup

1¾ oz (50g) cacao powder

2 vanilla pods, cut in half lengthways or 1 teaspoon of vanilla powder.

1   Toast the hazelnuts in a hot oven at approximately 350°F (170°C) for 10–15 minutes and pour out onto a thick, dry tea towel. Rub off as many of the skins as possible and pour them into a high-powered blender.
2   Blend to form a thick paste which will take approximately 10 minutes.
3   In the meantime melt the cacao butter or coconut oil in a bowl placed over a pan of boiling water. Once melted remove from the heat and stir in the vanilla, sweetener and cacao powder until you have a smooth consistency.
4   With the motor still running on the hazelnut butter, slowly add the chocolate mixture a little at a time and allow it to blend in before you add more. Taste and add 1–2 more tablespoons of maple syrup if needed.
5   Scoop the nut butter into a small sterilised jar with a tight-sealing lid. Store in the fridge for up to one month (see the note on nut butter shelf life on page 31).

TIP: See the note on page 30 on sterilising jars.
    If you like a crunchy texture, pulse in some raw cacao nibs or extra hazelnuts at the end to give it a bit more bite.

MIXED BERRY CHIA JAM

1   Allow the frozen berries to thoroughly defrost for at least 1 hour before using.

2   Simmer the berries in a saucepan set over a medium heat with the water and lemon juice for about 20 minutes, until the berries have softened. Stir in the chia seeds, sweetener and vanilla extract.

3   If you like your jam smooth, use a hand-held blender or pour it into a blender and pulse the jam to your desired consistency. I like mine chunky so I skip this step, but I use a potato masher to mash any bigger berries.

4   Continue to cook for about 5 minutes to make sure the chia seeds are evenly mixed in. Taste it to ensure it's sweet enough, or if you would like it to be more tart, add a little more lemon juice, just a few drops at a time.

5   Pour into a sterilised jar with a tight-fitting lid (see the note on how to sterilise jars on page 30). Once the jar has cooled down, store the jam in the fridge for up to three weeks.

TIPS: If you like a sharp, sour taste, zest the lemon before you juice it and add a little to the jam along with the chia, sweetener and vanilla.

This is a great way of using fresh berries, but as there are no preservatives in this jam, it needs to be used up quite quickly and returned to the fridge as soon as possible between uses.

I avoided jam for a few years because I assumed that it was filled with too much sugar, but discovering this chia jam renewed my love of it. When I first made this, the smell immediately transported me back to my childhood. My family used to spend our summers in Brittas Bay, and one year we went berry picking but our eyes were definitely bigger than our tummies. With the berries starting to turn, my mum decided to make jam and the rich, sweet smell of berries and sugar filled the whole house. Soon she realised that we didn't have enough jars, so I went running around to the neighbours – the deal was that if they had a jam jar or suitable container, they would get it back filled with jam.

Makes 1 small jar

approx. 8¾ oz (250g) frozen mixed
    berries
2 tablespoons filtered water
1 tablespoon lemon juice
2 tablespoons chia seeds
2 tablespoons maple or agave syrup
½ teaspoon vanilla extract

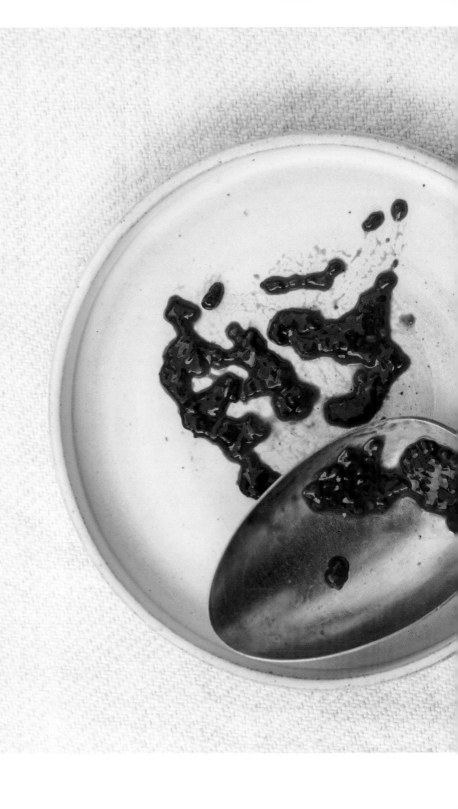

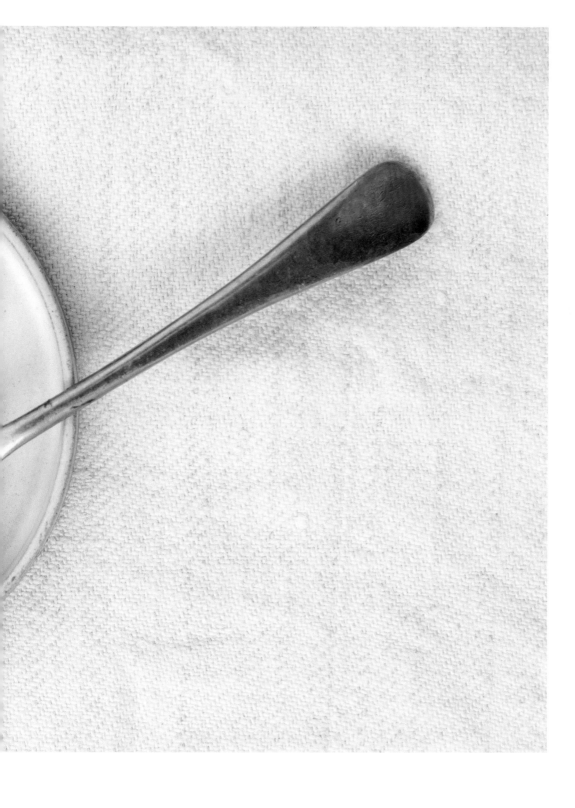

I always start my demonstrations by making almond milk. It's incredibly easy and making this most mornings takes just a few minutes. Making your own milk means you control what's in it and you can customise the sweetness.
I have also included some fruity options and the creamiest hot chocolate you will ever try!

NUT MILKS & DRINKS

VANILLA ALMOND MILK

With any nut milk, the ratio is 1:3 – one part soaked nuts to three parts water – if you want to scale this up.

You'll need a nut milk bag for this.

Makes approx. 3 cups (700ml)

5¼ oz (150g) almonds

approx. 3¼ cup (750ml) filtered water

1 tablespoon maple or brown
   rice syrup

1 teaspoon vanilla extract

a pinch of Himalayan pink salt or
   Maldon sea salt

1   Put the almonds in a bowl, cover with filtered water and soak for at least 8 hours or ideally overnight, then drain and rinse. (See the note on page 30 on soaking nuts.)

2   Put all the ingredients in a high-powered blender and blend on high for a minimum of 30 seconds. Strain through a nut milk bag and pour into a mason jar with a screw-top lid or a bottle with a tightly fitting lid.

3   Store in the fridge for up to three days. As it contains no stabilisers or additives it will separate naturally, but a quick shake solves that!

TIPS: You can find nut milk bags in health food stores. They're also called jam bags.

Feel free to adjust the sweetness to your liking or add some berries or fruits at the blending stage to make fruit milk, like the strawberry and mango milk on page 290.

You can use the leftover nut pulp to make the almond crackers on page 254.

CHOCOLATE MILK

1   Put the almonds in a bowl, cover with filtered water and soak for at least 8 hours or ideally overnight, then drain and rinse. (See the note on page 30 on soaking nuts.)

2   Put all the ingredients in a high-powered blender and blend on high for a minimum of 30 seconds. Strain through a nut milk bag and pour into a mason jar with a screw-top lid or a bottle with a tightly fitting lid.

3   Store in the fridge for up to three days. As it contains no stabilisers or additives it will separate naturally, but a quick shake solves that!

TIP: You can use your favourite sweetener in this, but using a liquid one means it blends easily so that you can quickly blend in a little more if required.

Sometimes it's the simple things in life that give the most pleasure. Chocolate milk is reminiscent of childhood and this vegan version is totally delicious.

You'll need a nut milk bag for this.

Makes approx. 3 cups (700ml)

5 oz (150g) almonds

approx. 3¼ cup (750ml) filtered
    water

1½ tablespoons maple or brown
    rice syrup

1 tablespoon raw cacao powder

1 teaspoon vanilla extract

a pinch of Himalayan pink salt or
    Maldon sea salt

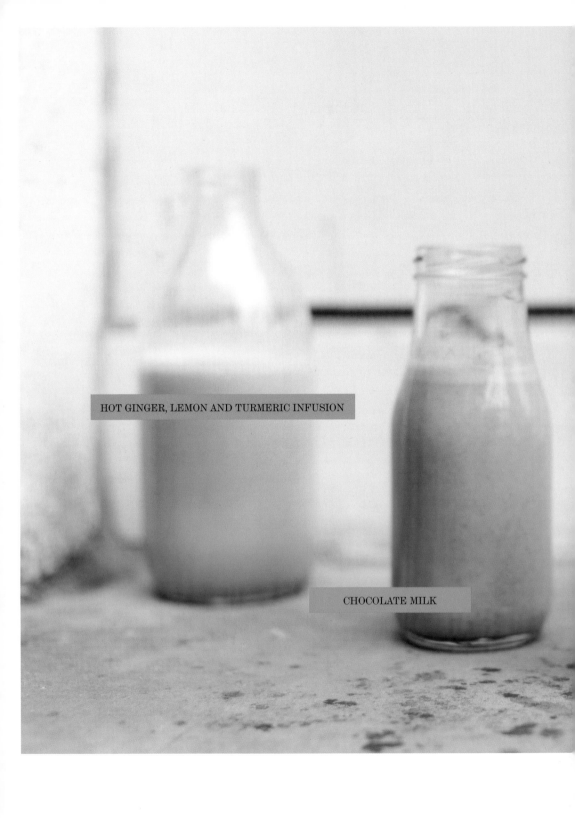

HOT GINGER, LEMON AND TURMERIC INFUSION

CHOCOLATE MILK

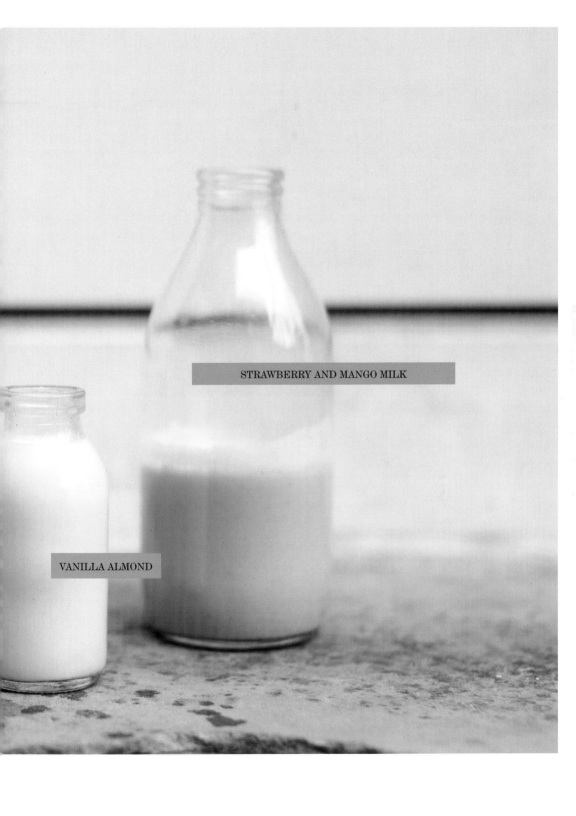

STRAWBERRY AND MANGO MILK

VANILLA ALMOND

STRAWBERRY AND MANGO MILK

The beauty of making your own milk is that you can flavour it easily and know exactly what's in it. When fruit is just about to turn it's at its sweetest and softest and injects lots of flavour into almond milk.

You'll need a nut milk bag for this.

Makes 3⅓ cups (800ml)

5¼ oz (150g) almonds

2 oz (60g) fresh strawberries, hulled, or frozen berries, thawed

2 oz (60g) fresh mango or 70g frozen mango pieces

3¼ cup (750ml) filtered water

1 tablespoon maple or brown rice syrup

1 teaspoon vanilla extract

1 teaspoon freeze-dried raspberry powder (optional)

a pinch of Himalayan pink salt or Maldon sea salt

1 Put the almonds in a bowl, cover with filtered water and soak for at least 8 hours or ideally overnight, then drain and rinse. (See the note on page 30 on soaking nuts.)

2 Put all the ingredients in a high-powered blender and blend on high for a minimum of 30 seconds. Strain through a nut milk bag and pour into a mason jar with a screw-top lid or a bottle with a tightly fitting lid.

3 Store in the fridge for up to three days. As it contains no stabilisers or additives it will separate naturally, but a quick shake solves that!

TIPS: Freeze-dried raspberry powder can be hard to find and isn't essential here, but it really gives it a kick.

Feel free to adjust the sweetness to your liking.

You can use the leftover nut pulp to make the almond crackers on page 254.

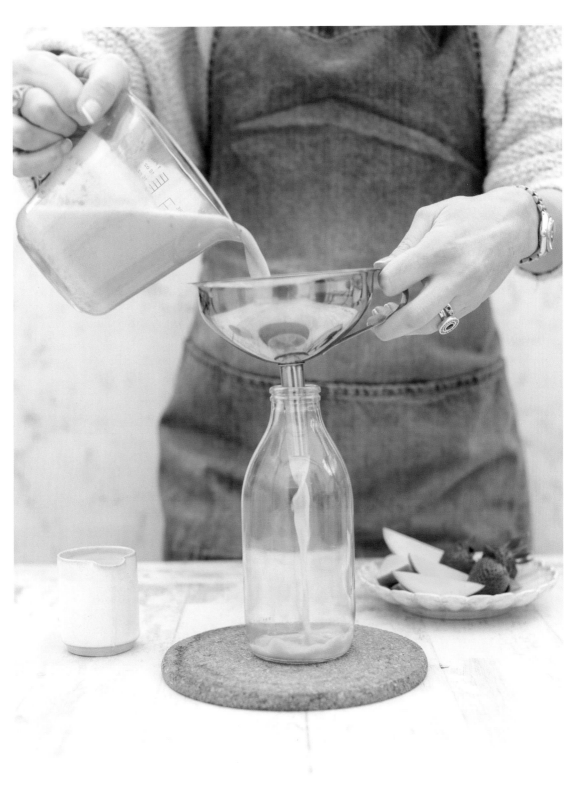

BRAZIL NUT, TURMERIC AND MACA MILK

This is creamy and delicious way to consume a lot of fresh raw turmeric, which has so many health benefits. But first, a word of warning: turmeric stains everything it touches – chopping boards, tea towels, your clothes – so use disposable kitchen paper to clean up any spills and do so immediately. It will also stain your nails, so try not to handle it too much once it's chopped.

You'll need a nut milk bag for this.

Makes approx. 1¼ cup (300ml)

2½ oz (70g) Brazil nuts

4 Medjool dates, pitted

1 x 2" (5cm) piece of fresh turmeric, scrubbed

1 vanilla pod, cut in half lengthways and seeds scraped out

approx. 1¼ cup (300ml) filtered water

1 teaspoon maca powder (optional)

¼ teaspoon coconut oil, ideally cold-pressed extra virgin organic

a pinch of Himalayan pink salt

1   Put the Brazil nuts in a bowl, cover with filtered water and soak for at least 8 hours or ideally overnight, then drain and rinse. (See the note on page 30 on soaking nuts.)

2   Put all the ingredients in a high-powered blender and blend on high for a minimum of 30 seconds. Strain through a nut milk bag and pour into a mason jar with a screw-top lid or a bottle with a tightly fitting lid.

3   Store in the fridge for up to three days. As it contains no stabilisers or additives it will separate naturally, but a quick shake solves that!

TIPS: Wash your blender immediately or the next thing you make will have a yellow tinge!

This can be gently warmed, but I like it at room temperature, ideally straight after making it.

You can substitute any other nut or seed for the Brazil nuts in this recipe.

HOT GINGER, LEMON AND TURMERIC INFUSION

1 Pour everything into a small saucepan and simmer gently for 6–8 minutes before straining into a warmed mug. Taste and feel free to dilute it with a little more water or add more sweetener.

TIPS: Turmeric stains everything it touches – chopping boards, tea towels, your clothes – so don't use anything to prepare this that you don't want to be stained yellow for the rest of its life, and use disposable kitchen paper to clean up any spills immediately. It will also stain your nails, so try not to handle it too much once it's grated.

A warmed mug will keep your hot drinks warmer for longer. Allow the kettle to half boil, then fill your mug with the hot water. Leave it to stand while you make the infusion and pour out the water when it's ready.

Inspired by a cold that took me by surprise during an incredibly busy time at work and wouldn't leave for a month, this is a punchy but effective infusion.

Serves 1

1 cup (250ml) filtered water
juice of ½ lemon
1 teaspoon grated fresh ginger
1 teaspoon grated fresh turmeric
1 teaspoon maple or agave syrup
1/8 teaspoon cayenne pepper

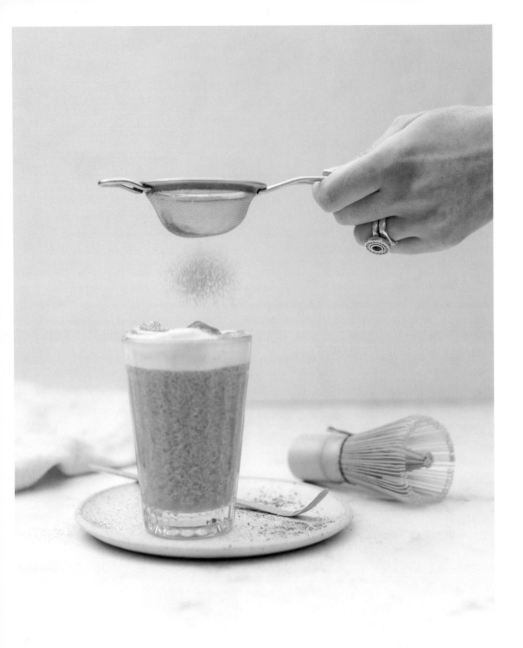

MATCHA AND CINNAMON LATTE

1   Pour your plant-based milk into a small saucepan and gently warm it. Matcha is renowned for its beneficial properties but it's important to never boil it, as that depletes the nutrients.

2   Put the matcha powder in a bowl with half of the water. Using the whisk that came with the tea or the back of a teaspoon, stir to blend the powder and water into a thick paste, pressing any clumps of powder with the back of the spoon to break them up. When fully blended, add the remaining water and the coconut oil and whisk again.

3   If you have a hand-held frother, use that on your milk now to create some foam.

4   Pour the matcha into a heated mug and pour the foamy milk on top. Drizzle with the agave syrup, dust with cinnamon and enjoy.

TIPS: I highly recommend picking up a little hand-held frother. I have an Aerolatte and it works really well.

A warmed mug will keep your hot drinks warmer for longer. Allow the kettle to half boil, then fill your mug with the hot water. Leave it to stand while you make your latte and pour out the water when it's ready.

I decided to swap coffee for matcha tea this year. I don't know how long that will last, but to distract me from the gorgeous aroma of coffee brewing, I knew I had to find a way to make matcha more appetising, which is where this matcha and cinnamon latte comes in.

Serves 1

3⅓ fl oz (100ml) plant-based milk

½ teaspoon powdered matcha tea

3⅓ fl oz (100ml) just-boiled water

½ teaspoon coconut oil

1 teaspoon agave syrup

a pinch of ground cinnamon

THE CREAMIEST HOT CHOCOLATE

This hot chocolate would easily rival the traditional variety and is a brilliant way to convince non-vegans that you're not completely crazy for eating this way!

Serves 1

1 cup (250ml) plant-based milk (or just fill the mug you'll be using with milk and use that as your measure)

1 tablespoon agave syrup, plus extra to taste

1 tablespoon almond butter

1 tablespoon raw cacao powder

1 teaspoon lucuma powder (optional)

a spoonful of vanilla coconut cream (page 309), to serve (optional)

1   Blend the milk, agave syrup, almond butter, cacao powder and lucuma powder together. It will likely need more sweetener, so taste it, add a little more agave and blend again, adding more if needed.

2   Transfer to a small saucepan set over a medium-low heat. Stir gently and ensure it doesn't boil or overheat. It will thicken up, like custard.

3   Serve in a warmed mug with a little vanilla coconut cream on top (if using).

TIPS: The lucuma powder is optional, but it adds a nice caramel taste.

To make this even more decadent you could melt some chocolate over it and add cacao nibs for a little texture.

A warmed mug will keep your hot drinks warmer for longer. Allow the kettle to half boil, then fill your mug with the hot water. Leave it to stand while you make your hot chocolate and pour out the water when it's ready.

To take this in a completely different direction, skip heating the milk, add a shot of espresso and pour it over ice for an iced mocha.

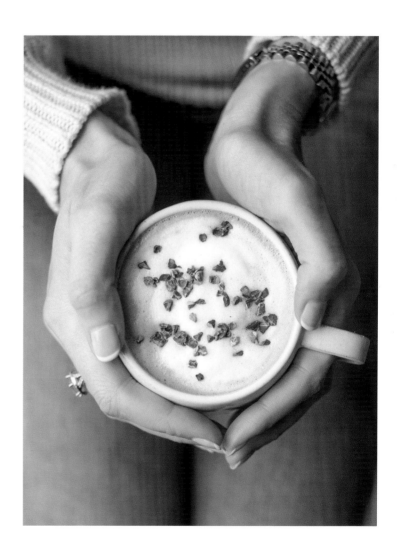

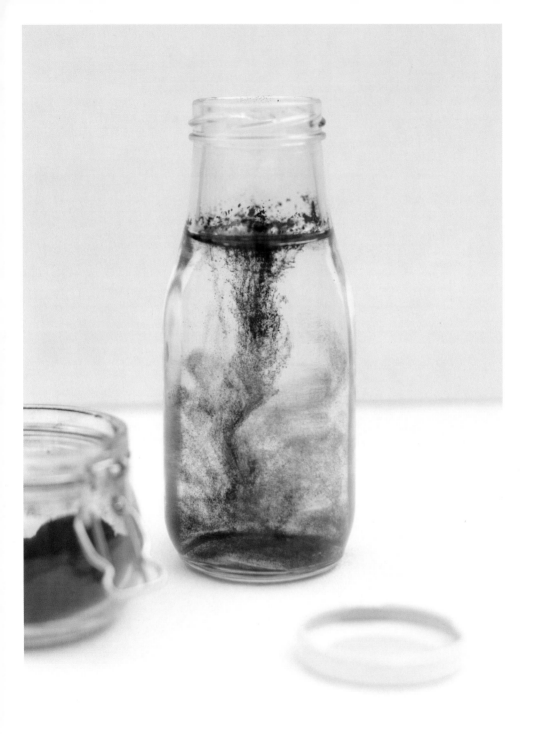

CHARCOAL AND CHIA DETOX WATER

1 Put the water, chia and charcoal in a 4¼-cup (1-litre) water bottle and squeeze in the lemon juice before adding the whole wedge too. Put on the lid and shake to combine.

TIP: Charcoal in powdered form can get very messy, so be careful!

This almost seems too simple to put in a cookbook, but whenever I put a photo of this on my Instagram feed I get asked lots of questions about it. I drink this first thing in the morning. You might be surprised at how full you feel after drinking this, as chia seeds have lots of fibre.

I bought activated charcoal from a market stall and started reading up on it. It has been used as a detox agent for centuries, for filtering both water and air. You will likely have seen it in beauty products too, as it's used in whitening toothpastes and face masks.

While activated charcoal has been proven to be beneficial at removing bacteria and toxins from your body, you shouldn't use it on a daily basis if you're ingesting it. I might have this a few times a month, but no more.

Serves 1

approx. 2 cup (500ml) filtered water
½ teaspoon chia seeds (ground or whole seeds both work)
¼ teaspoon activated charcoal
1 lemon wedge

I'm a big believer in the fact that sometimes simple things done well are all you need. This chapter is testament to that and is filled with a few simple additions that are really worthwhile to master. Whether it's making your own stock, cooking quinoa perfectly, lentils done just right or whipping up a silky smooth caramel sauce, all the details are in here.

STAPLES

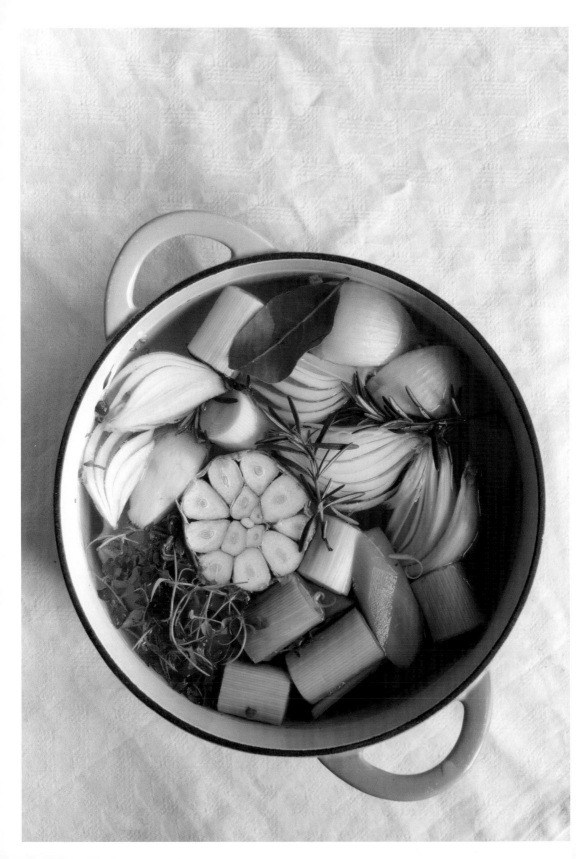

VEGETABLE STOCK

1   Put all the ingredients in a large pot with a lid or in a slow cooker. If you're cooking this on the hob, bring to the boil, then reduce the heat and simmer for anything from 2 to 6 hours depending on how strong and concentrated you want the flavour to be. If you're using a slow cooker it will take at least 4 hours on a high heat, but you can leave it for up to 24 hours on a medium heat for a greater depth of flavour.

2   Strain through a sieve and use immediately or store in the fridge in an airtight container for up to three days. You can also freeze stock in airtight plastic containers – just run the container under the warm tap to help it release.

TIPS: The recipe works well as written, but go with what you have. You can use onion and garlic skins, the ends of carrots, celery bases and any fresh herbs you have – thyme works particularly well, as the warm water really pulls the flavour out.

Blend the stock with a small handful of soaked almonds or Brazil nuts for a creamy texture.

This can be added to lightly sautéed vegetables for a simple chunky vegetable soup or blend it if you would prefer a creamed soup.

I learned a really useful tip for making stock from Louise Hay, author of *You Can Heal Your Life*. She said she put a plastic bag in her freezer and over the course of a week added any vegetable cuttings she had to it. The freezing preserved them, and when she was ready to make stock it was simply a case of cooking them up. I now do this and it amazes me how quickly the bag fills up, not to mention that having everything already chopped up makes this incredibly simple to prepare.

Makes 4¼ cups (1 litre)

7 carrots, roughly chopped

3 onions, roughly chopped

2 celery sticks, roughly chopped

1 leek, roughly chopped

2 garlic cloves, peeled and left whole

1 small sprig of fresh thyme

1 small sprig of fresh rosemary

1 bay leaf

4¼ cup (1 litre) filtered water

TOMATO SAUCE

This is so versatile and turns pasta, brown rice and vegetables into something special.

Serves 4

1 tablespoon olive oil

1 large onion, finely chopped

3 garlic cloves, crushed

2 x 14 oz (400g) tins of chopped
    tomatoes

1 sprig of fresh thyme

½ teaspoon dried oregano

a pinch of sugar

sea salt and freshly ground
    black pepper

fresh basil, to garnish (optional)

1   Heat the oil in a saucepan set over a medium heat. Add the onion and garlic and fry for 8 minutes, until lightly golden. Add the tomatoes, thyme, oregano and sugar. Reduce the heat to low and simmer for 20–30 minutes, stirring occasionally, until the sauce has reduced and thickened. Remove the thyme sprig and discard. Season to taste with salt and pepper and garnish with fresh basil (if using) to serve.

2   This will keep in an airtight container in the fridge for up to five days. It also freezes well, so it's worth making a double batch and freezing half.

CASHEW CHEESE

1 Put the cashews in a bowl, cover with filtered water and soak for at least 8 hours or ideally overnight. Drain and rinse, then pat them dry thoroughly with a clean tea towel or kitchen paper. (See the note on page 30 on soaking nuts.)

2 Put the soaked cashews in a blender along with the nutritional yeast, miso, lemon juice, a pinch of salt and a little just-boiled water, using the plunger to ensure it all gets blended evenly. Drizzle in more water until it's a smooth consistency similar to hummus. Scoop it out into a serving bowl, then drizzle the olive oil over the top and scatter over the paprika.

3 This can be stored in an airtight container in the fridge for up to a week if you have leftovers.

TIP: Use white miso to maintain the creamy colour of the cashew cheese.

Cashew cheese is a nice introduction to vegan cheeses, plus it's really versatile and can be used for lots of things. I like to serve it with baked sweet potatoes (page 107) or wedges (page 174).

Makes 4 portions

5¼ oz (150g) cashew nuts

2 tablespoons nutritional yeast

1½ teaspoons white miso paste

1 teaspoon lemon juice

a pinch of sea salt

just-boiled water, as needed

1 tablespoon olive oil

pinch of paprika

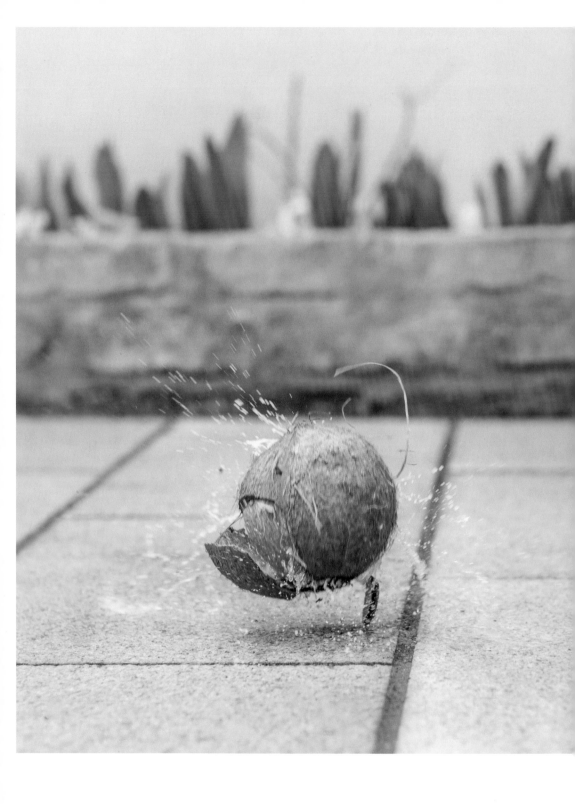

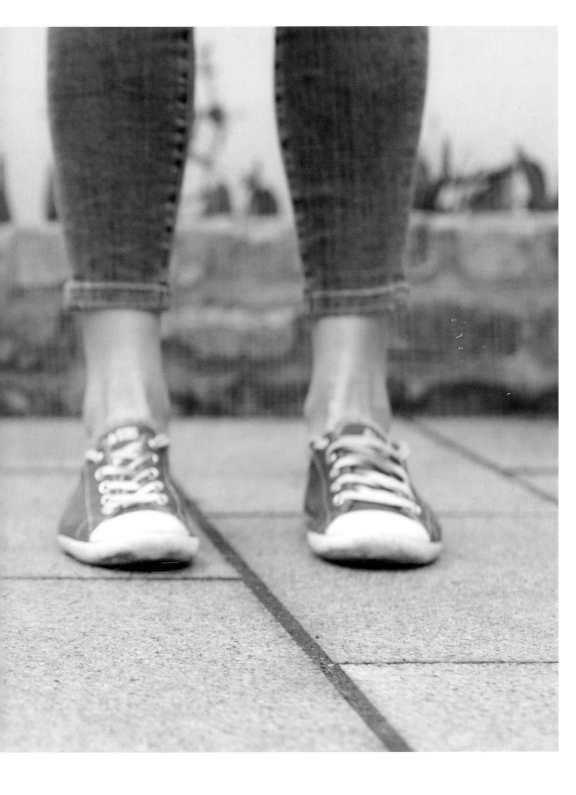

COCONUT CREAM

You'll notice that lots of recipes in this book call for the coconut cream that you find at the top of a tin of coconut milk. Here's the foolproof way to separate the cream from the water so that you can easily scoop it out.

Makes 6 tablespoons

1 x approx. 1¾ cup (400ml) tin of full-fat coconut milk

1   Put the tin of coconut milk in the fridge for at least 1 hour, but ideally overnight. Take the chilled tin out of the fridge without shaking it. Open the tin and turn it upside down to drain out the water into a bowl and set this aside. Use a spatula to scoop out the creamy top layer, making sure you get every last bit to use as needed.

TIP: Don't throw out the coconut water after you've scooped out the cream – save it for adding to smoothies, soups, casseroles or desserts.

VANILLA COCONUT CREAM

1 To make the vanilla coconut cream, you need to put the tin of coconut milk in the fridge for at least 1 hour, or ideally overnight. Put a medium-sized bowl in the fridge or freezer to chill it too.

2 Take the tin of coconut milk out of the fridge without shaking it. Open the tin and turn it upside down to drain out the water into a bowl and set this aside. Use a spatula to scoop out the creamy top layer into your chilled bowl, making sure you get every last bit.

3 Working quickly, whisk the cream, agave and vanilla together to form a thick paste. Don't over-whip or you will melt the coconut cream and it will collapse.

4 This will keep in the fridge in an airtight container for up to five days.

TIPS: Don't throw out the coconut water after you've scooped out the cream – save it for adding to smoothies, soups, casseroles or desserts.

I use light agave, which keeps the cream a nice pale colour. If you use dark agave or a date or maple syrup it will still taste delicious, but the colour will be a little yellow.

To make this into a lemon coconut cream, add the zest of 1 lemon along with the agave syrup and vanilla.

Whipped coconut cream is a bit of a revelation. The first time I had it, I realised I'd been missing that creamy texture with desserts. There's no need to go without it ever again!

Makes 6¾ fl oz (200ml) or 4 servings

1 x approx. 1¾ cup (400ml) tin of full-fat coconut milk

1 teaspoon light agave syrup

½ teaspoon vanilla powder or 1 vanilla pod, cut in half lengthways and seeds scraped out

CARAMEL SAUCE

This vegan caramel sauce will amaze you, as it's so quick to make and so delicious. It instantly elevates simple things like yogurt or a fruit crumble to a whole different level. I love to dip dark chocolate in this, pour some over a bowl of fruit or drizzle grilled pineapple wedges with it (see page 214).

Makes 1 small jar

approx. 12 oz (350g) Medjool dates, pitted
4 tablespoons coconut cream from a tin (see page 308)
1 tablespoon maple syrup
2 tablespoons melted coconut oil
1 vanilla pod, cut in half lengthways and seeds scraped out, or ¼ teaspoon vanilla powder
a pinch of sea salt

1   Blend the dates in a food processor, then add the coconut cream and maple syrup and blend again. With the motor running, drizzle in the melted coconut oil. Add the vanilla and a pinch of salt at the end and pulse to combine.

TIP: Save the coconut water from the tin after scooping out the cream and use it to dilute the caramel sauce it if it's too thick.

LENTILS

1 Put the lentils and water in a large pot and bring to the boil. Cover tightly, then reduce the heat and simmer for 15–20 minutes, until they are tender. If you're using split red lentils, however, they typically take only 5–7 minutes to cook.

2 Season with salt after cooking – if salt is added before you cook them, the lentils will become tough.

3 Allow to cool, then store in an airtight container in the fridge for up to three days.

TIPS: Cook lentils in a 3:1 ratio of three parts water to one part lentils, so scale it up as needed.

Ensure your pot is big enough, as the lentils will triple in size.

I always add some vegan vegetable bouillon to the water.

Having cooked lentils to hand is a great way of quickly injecting plant-based protein into and bulking up salads, stews and soups. They have quite a neutral taste and absorb the flavours of whatever you add them to.

Lentils don't require soaking, unlike other pulses. Just rinse them with cold fresh water before boiling to remove any dust that may have settled on them.

Serves 2

7 oz (200g) green, black or brown lentils

3¼ cup (750ml) filtered water

a pinch of sea salt

QUINOA

The key step here that improves the flavour immeasurably is popping your quinoa. I know it sounds strange, but trust me on this! Toasting quinoa releases its gorgeous nutty flavour.

Serves 2

7 oz (200g) quinoa
1 teaspoon coconut oil
approx. 2 cup (500ml) filtered water

1   Soak the quinoa in a bowl of filtered water for 15 minutes. Drain it in a sieve and rinse it under the tap. Shake it thoroughly to remove as much of the water as possible.

2   Put the coconut oil into whatever pan you will be cooking the quinoa in – you need one that has a lid – and allow to melt over a medium-high heat. When the oil is hot, add the quinoa and stir it around. The water will evaporate and you will start to hear a popping sound. Keep an eye on it at this stage, as it can burn easily. If you feel it's too hot, remove the pan from the heat straight away and shake the pan to distribute heat and prevent the quinoa from burning.

3   After about 2 minutes, when it's becoming lightly golden, add the filtered water and reduce the heat to medium-low. Simmer, covered, for 15–20 minutes, until all the water has evaporated and the quinoa is cooked. Turn off the heat, then put a clean tea towel or a piece of kitchen paper between the pot and the lid and leave it to sit for 5 minutes.

4   Allow to cool, then store in an airtight container in the fridge for up to three days.

TIPS: The ratio for cooking quinoa is two parts water to one part quinoa, so scale it up as needed.

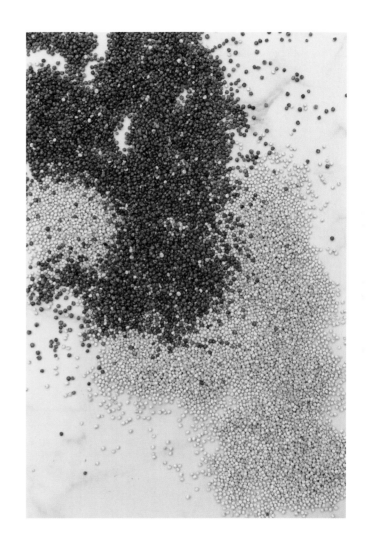

ACKNOWLEDGEMENTS

It's surreal to come to this stage of a book, when the testing is done, the photos have been taken and the writing has been edited. This book contains the hard work of so many people who all formed the most fabulous team. First, thank you to Deirdre at Gill Books for taking a chance and nurturing and harnessing my enthusiasm. Thank you to the phenomenal photography, food prep and styling team of Leo, Charlotte and Aoife.

Thank you to Graham for your fantastic sense of design. Thank you to Kristin for dotting the Is and crossing the Ts and a lot more in between.

Thank you to Teresa and Ellen for being just as excited as me about getting *Going Vegan* out into the world and sharing the message.

Lastly, thank you to my family for nurturing my love of food and creativity and to my followers for your constant support.

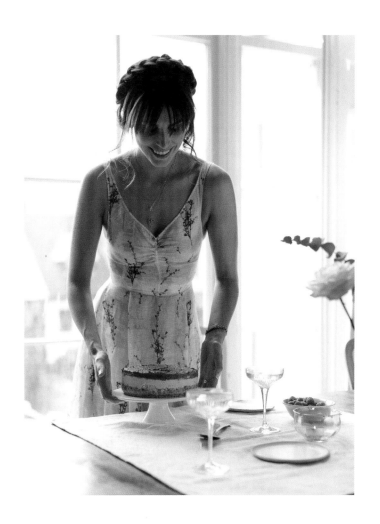

INDEX

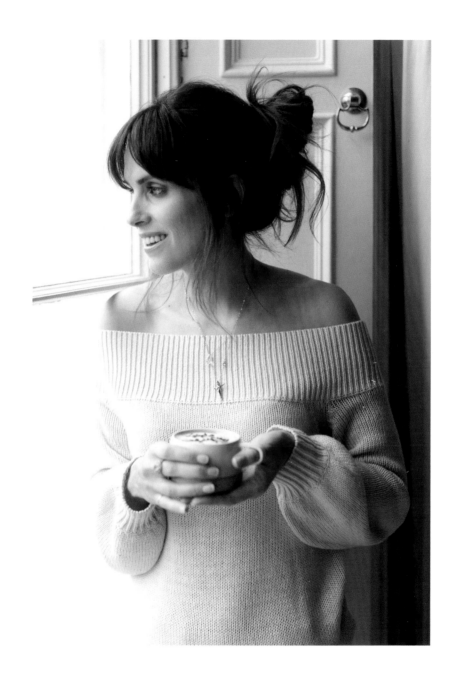